ROUTINE
MIRACLES

Personal Journeys
of Patients and Doctors
Discovering the Power
of Modern Medicine

ROUTINE

MIRACLES

CONRAD FISCHER, MD

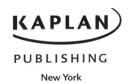

PUBLISHING

New York

© 2009 by Conrad Fischer, MD

Published by Kaplan Publishing, a division of Kaplan, Inc.
1 Liberty Plaza, 24th Floor
New York, NY 10006

Printed in the United States of America

10 9 8 7 6 5 4 3 2 1

Library of Congress Cataloging-in-Publication Data has been applied for.

Kaplan Publishing books are available at special quantity discounts to use for sales promotions, employee premiums, or educational purposes. Please email our Special Sales Department to order or for more information at *kaplanpublishing@ kaplan.com,* or write to Kaplan Publishing, 1 Liberty Plaza, 24th Floor, New York, NY 10006.

Dedicated to Father John Collins,
who helped me reach through the clouds of
unknowing for a higher, uniting vision of bringing
optimism and faith to a suffering humanity
on walks through the streets of New York City

CONTENTS

PREFACE

FOR 20 YEARS FATHER John Collins and I have walked the streets of New York together and, regardless of our destination, John has continually showered his best understanding of the grace of God on the people of this city, always showering just a little extra on police officers. When John was a little boy, his father, a New York City cop, died of a heart attack. My father, too, was a New York City cop, so there is always a squeeze on my left ventricle when I see John working with the police.

John and I walk and talk and try to decipher the meaning of the universe. We try to figure out the big questions: If there is a compassionate God, why is there suffering on the earth? How can bad accidents and disease happen to good people who pray and try to live right? We consider it a hobby: trying to pierce the mystery of existence and bring help to a suffering humanity. John also feeds me, a lot. Most of the home-cooked lunches I have had have been in the kitchen of the rectory of the Paulist Fathers on 58th Street in Manhattan.

John is over six feet tall, over 200 pounds—a big guy with a big beard and a happy smile. While he opens up a walk-in refrigerator, we continue our discussion of suffering and divine love.

We discuss the question of suffering and divine love. How can an all-powerful divinity that is said to be simultaneously all loving, leave us to pain and disease? I understand it better now that I have children. I cannot shield them from every injury. If my son falls and breaks his arm, I am sorry with him. If he becomes sick, it is not because I do not love him or care for him. Quite the opposite. When a child is ill, the parent is even more heartbroken than the child is. That is the way the universe is set up. After the act of creation, our children are separate from us. We can send them messages, but ultimately we cannot force them to think in a certain way. I believe such is the relationship of God to us. If we are injured, then God's heart is broken even before ours is. If another kid does an injustice to my child, then I am angry. But I cannot walk down the street and punch that kid in the face. Such is God's love, too: the love is always there, but the intervention cannot happen in the way the we might want it.

When people are sick, they are often sad and depressed. They are angry and frustrated. A faithful person may feel even more anger than a nonbelieving person. My father, an atheist, does not feel abandoned. My mother, a believer, feels heartbroken that God allowed her son, my brother, to be taken from her.

John and I have a remarkable similarity in our professional lives. An enormous part of our separate roles in life (his in a parish mission, mine in a board review class) is to liven up the joint, so to speak. The book you are reading was conceived on one of our strolls. It began as an exploration of a series of questions: If doctors can cure more people, relieve more suffering, than ever before, why aren't they suffused with an optimism that has them sprinting toward the next cure or breakthrough? If physicians have the highest salaries ever, with tremendous public trust, why do so many medical students — the majority, in fact, —think it was better to be in medicine 25 years ago? Now that we can do amazing science-fiction-type stuff for people, why aren't physicians more satisfied?

The book emerged as a collection of stories about the most remarkable medical advances in the last two decades, in the hope of creating a spiritual avalanche that will bury the negative attitudes weighing down doctors, medical students, and the general public. I think people will be more likely to find solutions to health care problems if they can take stock of all the fantastic things that have happened in medicine since the 1980s.

In the early part of that decade, John Collins was a 38-year-old priest. He exercised a lot, wanting to avoid his father's fate, but one day while take a swim after playing racquetball, he felt a twinge in his chest. "I knew something was happening," he says. "Then I did a dumb thing. I drove back to the rectory. I told another priest what was happening. He was smart enough to get me in the car and take me to the emergency department. I remember the clerk starting out with the 'What's your insurance?' question, when a nurse noticed that I was having chest pain and might be having a heart attack. I got taken in right away."

John was taken straight to the catheterization laboratory. A catheter is a thin plastic tube that goes in a blood vessel; in John's case, the catheter went into the coronary artery through the artery in his groin and revealed the presence of a blood clot. If there is a clot in the coronary artery, the heart dies.

And so do you.

The year was 1982. Doctors knew at the time that an aspirin would decrease a heart attack victim's risk of death by about 25 percent and that certain beta-blocker-type medications would decrease mortality by another 10 to 30 percent. There were also medications such as nitroglycerine and the old standard, morphine, to decrease the pain.

John was a lucky man that day. A doctor friend of his showed up at the lab. He told John about the clot-busting drugs for myocardial infarction (the medical term for heart attack) that were just then being studied. There was, the doctor said, an experimental protocol for a clot-busting medication, or thrombolytic, known as streptokinase. He would have to break the protocol, but he could get John the experimental drug.

John received the streptokinase about two hours after the start of his pain. The clot dissolved, flow to the myocardium was restored, and the myocardial infarction was stopped.

John, the priest and racquetball player, the erstwhile little boy whose father died of a heart attack, was snatched from the jaws of death by having the good fortune to live long enough to have his disease appear just as the first new clot-busting drug became available.

"My father had his heart attack in 1952," John says. "If he had lived in another time, when catheterization labs, thrombolytics like strepto-kinase, and angioplasty were available, he would have lived."

Can we take just a moment, just a second, please? To feel grateful. To feel fortunate.

Twelve years after his heart attack, John had an abnormal stress test. Blockages in the coronary arteries were choking off his heart. Such blockages, called stenoses (narrowings), result from cholesterol-filled plaques in the artery.

No problem, you say. Just another squirt of streptokinase and, zip, the plaques will melt away. Nope. Streptokinase and all versions of thrombolytic medications work only on acute blockages from clots. Myocardial infarctions happen when an atherosclerotic plaque ruptures and a new clot forms. At the end of the day, heart attacks are a clotting disorder. What to do about slowly progressive atherosclerotic plaques is another story.

What to offer? The latest thing in 1994 was to widen the artery, a process called angioplasty, and insert a metal tube or scaffolding called a stent. The stent pushes back the atherosclerotic, fibrofatty, lipid-laden clog in the artery. When deployed, it will stay open in about two-thirds of patients in the original version. Stenting had just been developed.

Another save just in the nick of time.

By this time, in addition to aspirin, a new antiplatelet medication known as clopidogrel had been developed. Combined with aspirin, it lowered the risk of the stent closing up from about 30 percent to about 20 to 25 percent.

That risk was still high. We can now, in 2009 as this book is going to press, coat the stent with a substance to prevent another clot. One of the greatest new advances in cardiology is understanding that plaques and disease in the coronary artery intersect with the immune system. Suppressing white cells like lymphocytes actually helps open the arteries, so coating the stent with an immunosuppressive agent, and thereby inhibiting lymphocytes, will help keep the stent open.

On an island in the Pacific, far from anything else, lies a remote place with giant stone sculptures of heads. Where did they come from? How did they get there? It is an enormous mystery. On this mysterious island, someone reaches down and takes a sample of soil. Under a microscope, the soil is found to contain a substance that, oddly enough, inhibits T cells (white blood cells that normally defend the body against infection) and is thus a selective immunosuppressive agent. It is derived from the bacterium *Streptomyces hygroscopicus*.

Easter Island is known to the natives as Rapa Nui. In honor of this name, the immunosuppressive agent in the island's soil is dubbed rapamycin. We use it topically to control psoriasis. We use it to prevent organ transplant rejection. We use it to prevent the rejection of bone marrow transplantation. And we use it to coat stents.

Since receiving his stent, Father John Collins has been around the world on his parish missions, preaching and being nice to the cops. He has outlived his father by more than 20 years.

Luck? Science? Mysterious head sculptures on Easter Island? Take your pick. Probably coincidence.

While he was on the operating table, with the catheter piercing his groin, the attending cardiologist suddenly recognized her patient. "You're Father Collins from the church next door! I go there for mass all the time. I know you! Say, listen, Father, I am three months pregnant. Will you baptize my baby?"

John remembers thinking, *Listen, sweetheart, if you get me out of here alive, I will put the kid through college for you.*

What he said was "Of course I'll do the baptism."

Six months later, a pain-free, fully alive Father Collins held the baby in his arms.

Another stent, another baptism.

Another day to hang out with your friend and decipher the meaning of love in the universe.

—CONRAD FISCHER, MD

ROUTINE
MIRACLES

PART I

Practicing Alchemy on the Streets of New York

CHAPTER I

The Heart of the Matter

Physician Dissatisfaction and How to Cure It

"PUT ON YOUR HELMET, and remember the sweat that poured off you in summer practice! You are the best! You are winners! Now act like it and knock those guys off the field!" our high school football coach would say. If we'd lost against the opposing team the year before, he would remind us: "You've done a lot of work since last year. You are not the same individuals, the same team you were before. You have grown. You are the best team we ever put out there. Today belongs to you!"

I can't imagine any sports team succeeding at any level with a coach saying, "You're weak and wimpy compared to me when I played the game. You're not as good as my teammates were! And, most of all, you won't enjoy the game as much as we did 25 years ago. Now go out there and take a beating!" Yet if medical school faculty were football coaches, this is exactly what they would sound like.

There is a chorus of older physicians' voices that is having an unhealthy sway over medical students. "Has anyone here been told you are the best, better than the faculty?" I ask a class of mine. No hands go up. "Has anyone here been told you are worse than students in the past, that you are not as diligent, devoted, or hardworking?" Eighty percent of the hands go up. Eighty percent of my students have been actively discouraged by their "coaches"—and just look who is playing for the other team: cancer, diabetes, heart disease, stroke, rheumatoid arthritis, AIDS, psoriasis, reflux disease, fibroids, epilepsy, kidney disease, and loss of hearing, sight, limbs, and spirit. Talk about a formidable opponent!

Dr. Sheldon Landesman, the assistant dean of education at SUNY Downstate Medical Center in Brooklyn, New York, is one of those "coaches." Sheldon graduated from medical school more than 35 years ago. He is a tall man in his early sixties with graying hair and a quick wit. I have known Sheldon for more than 10 years. He is good-natured and actually quite devoted to his students, but he gives them the distinct feeling, not indirectly, that medical students of his generation were more committed, more studious, and more serious than students today are.

Sheldon and I both did our internships in the years before the death of a young woman named Libby Zion in a New York City emergency department led to the regulation of duty hours in training. When we were on call, we were in the hospital for 24 to 36 hours at a stretch. Going without sleep for so long, we had the same judgment levels and psychomotor skills as if we were legally drunk. But internships had been structured like that for the past hundred years; long duty hours were a rite of passage that lent a Superman mystique to the profession.

Interns now can work no more than 24 hours at a time, no more than 80 hours a week. Despite the effects that sleep deprivation has on performance, many thought leaders in medicine, including Sheldon, bemoan the degradation in training that they feel comes with duty-hour limits. "Where is the continuity of care? Where is the devotion to your profession and medicine?" they ask. "Don't you want Iron Man to take care of you, not just some ordinary citizen who needs to sleep eight hours before he can do your bypass surgery?"

Even I still feel macho about the long hours I worked during my internship. I mention it every chance I get, followed by an exposition on the dangers of sleep deprivation. If I were a veteran, I'd be saying, "War is hell; all war should stop. Now let me tell you what I did in the war."

Duty-hour limits are only part of the mentor generation's complaint. When I ask Sheldon for his help on the research project on which this book is based, he jumps to my side. Sheldon is an exemplar of academic productivity and research activity. He has repeatedly won million-dollar National Institutes of Health grants, becoming over the years the most well-funded researcher in the Department of Medicine at SUNY Downstate Medical Center. He is single-handedly responsible for one-fifth of the entire curriculum in the second year of medical school.

"What are you studying?" he asks.

I explain to him that I am examining why many of our students, residents, and physicians think that our profession was better 25 years ago. Not only do I want my students to become clinician-scientists devoted to finding cures, but I also want them to recognize that they are at the peak of civilization, the top 1 percent in intelligence, education, experience, and capabilities.

"They can accomplish anything they set their minds to," I say. "I want them to feel this, and I want to know why they don't feel it."

Sheldon says, "Because it is not true."

"What?" I ask him.

"Medicine *was* better before."

"But, Sheldon," I say, "that doesn't make sense." I start to remind him about the things doctors can do now that people once thought you had to be a biblical figure to accomplish—restore sight and hearing, fix broken hearts, make arthritis patients walk, end epileptic seizures, even cure some cancers.

Sheldon, seeing things from a doctor's point of view, not the patient's, stops me short. "Medicine is worse now. It is less satisfying."

What, then, are the sources of doctors' dissatisfaction?

"In the past," Sheldon says, "the doctor was in charge. We had autonomy. We controlled things."

Autonomy is a big issue for the older generation. In the course of conducting interviews for this book, I meet Dr. Erick Lang, who performed the world's first angiogram of the coronary arteries in 1959 and remains at the cutting edge of interventional radiology. I ask him why he thinks so many students and young physicians say things were better 25 years ago.

"It has always been this way," he responds. "There is always the feeling that your golden days are always behind you. In 1959, they told me it was better 25 years before that."

I ask him why we are not more satisfied with medicine, considering how much more we can do in treatment.

"Now new advances are done by whole teams of investigators," he says. "There is less personal glory. When one man did the work before, it gave a greater feeling of accomplishment. The sense of personal satisfaction has been removed."

Another area where the older generation feels its autonomy is threatened is patient empowerment. We are entering an age where it's possible again for doctors and patients to have a dialogue, thanks largely to the Internet, which allows patients to research their diseases and follow up at the doctor's office with intelligent questions. Yet many senior physicians lament their lost status; they either don't realize or don't care that it is through patient empowerment that patient trust has risen to an all-time high.

Doctors are devoted as ever. The commitment of physicians to the art of medicine and to humanity is not in question. When asked whether they would still practice medicine if they did not have to work for a living, 80 percent of respondents said yes. That is devotion! But the irritations and complexities of our current method of practice sorely test that devotion. Physician income is high, but not high enough to compensate for the difficulties of practice.

Sheldon brings up another point: "Medical students are graduating with phenomenal amounts of debt. How do you expect them to choose some altruistic practice or clinician-scientist job and be saddled with this for decades to come?"

Much of the reason for physician dissatisfaction despite greater treatment breakthroughs is related to how we finance medical school education. Student debt is a huge barrier to a young graduate's pursuit of a career in research or primary care. For years, 25 percent of a typical graduate's income will go toward repaying student loans, sometimes amounting to hundreds of thousands of dollars.

At the same time, faculty at medical schools have seen drastic cuts in financial support for their research and teaching. To make a living, these clinician-scientists are compelled to see patients in private practice while also fulfilling their duties as teachers. This is a serious defect in the system.

If Americans want to expect top-notch medical care in the coming decades, the public must act now to reform the financing of medical education. Faculty need financial freedom to teach and to continue to do the kind of research that has made the United States the world's most technologically brilliant society. Faculty have grown increasingly angry and resentful of greater work with less support, and students are turning away in droves from research and primary care.

Sheldon Landesman points out that students want easier specialties. "In 1972, when I graduated," he says, "the best and brightest went into internal medicine. Now they want dermatology, radiology, and emergency medicine. All of these specialties are lifestyle specialties. The hours are controlled. The responsibilities are limited."

Do we want the best and brightest of our society to pursue medical research? Or do we want them merely to be clearing up acne and performing standard X-rays?

Before we can answer those questions, we must address one more issue related to doctors' dissatisfaction, one that is bound up with the issues of autonomy and financial constraints: health insurance companies.

"Everything is controlled by the insurance companies," Sheldon Landesman says.

"Sheldon," I reply, "in 1968, the year you entered school, 93 percent of health care expenditures were out of pocket. Now 85 percent are from third-party payers, insurers. Isn't that better?" I ask.

"That is the problem," he answers. "We are not free to do what we think is right."

To say that students identify dealing with health insurance companies as problematic is an understatement. When asked about their least satisfying, most painful experience, 92 percent of physicians and students agreed or strongly agreed that dealing with insurance companies made medicine less satisfying and less attractive to practice. Put another way, only 8 percent did not feel that the single greatest source of dissatisfaction in medicine was the health insurance industry. Society and our government will ignore this fact at their own peril.

Students who get accepted into medical school are in the top 10 percent of their college class. These are people who have options. We must make medicine more satisfying and attractive for them. If we want the best and brightest to see healing people as the most desirable thing to do with their talents, the obstacles of fighting with insurance companies must be fixed. We should not every year see a fight in Congress to prevent a reduction in hospital reimbursements. We should not have to save Medicare in a last-minute rescue.

It is my sincere hope that the United States will soon provide universal health insurance coverage for all its citizens. In the 1960s, physicians were actually opposed to the Medicare system because of the fear of this scary thing called socialized medicine. Even in the 1990s, when there was a major push to have universal coverage, physicians were still resistant. But now, however, the medical profession has come around to the fact that we must achieve the goal of insuring all U.S. citizens. U.S. physicians, their major professional groups, and their academic leadership are now on board.

DR. SHELDON LANDESMAN and I agree on some things. Doctors today face formidable obstacles in their practice. They are having to fight cancer, heart disease, stroke, and so on, and at the same time deal with managed care, lack of insurance, fear of malpractice, debt, and the demands of a family. As a result, many more students than in the past choose specialties where these problems are not as likely to affect their work. They are giving up on research, which just doesn't pay. The best and brightest are deciding to pursue dermatology instead of tackling diabetes.

Meanwhile, their teachers are making it easier for them to make such decisions by saying the equivalent of "You're so weak and whiny, you'd never cure diabetes anyway."

This is where I part ways with Sheldon. Sure, it's difficult to practice today. Managed care is the bane of my existence. But that's all the more reason to celebrate our students, to give them encouragement in the face of all these obstacles, to say to them not that the profession is at its nadir because we have lost our machismo to duty-hour limits, our autonomy to teamwork and patient empowerment, and our freedom to financial burdens and insurance companies, but rather that this is actually medicine's finest hour because we are making advances at exponential rates. Rather than teach students to complain, resist change, and blindly follow authority, we should be teaching them to keep an open mind at all times. That is the way to have hope. By being open-minded and creative, doctors can again find satisfaction in their work. I want to get to the bottom of all the narrow-mindedness, because I want more students to be physician-scientists who fight over the best research positions rather than the highest-paid positions. I want them not to have to worry about money for loan repayment, so that they can choose a life of investigation and medical discovery as physician-scientists, academic doctors. I want the main goal of our students to be eradicating disease, not finding an easy, high-paying job in a subspecialty. I think if we tell students, "You are the most knowledgeable, most expert people ever to leave our doors," it would give them the audacity to feel that things like curing cancer and getting universal health insurance are possible.

I want to restore my students' faith and hope in medicine by showing them all the amazing things their predecessors have done, not for the sake of celebrating their predecessors, but to inspire them to go beyond even those remarkable advances. I want students to feel blessed that they can raise the dead, restore sight to the blind, restore hearing to the deaf, and cure leprosy for $1.59. I want them to feel blessed to have patients who are grateful and well-informed. But how can they be aware of these blessings when faculty members, their role models, are selling them on the idea that it is worse to be in the profession compared with 25 years ago?

I tell my students, "Many of you are smarter than I am. I may be more knowledgeable than you are now, because I have more experience, and I have been doing it longer, but that does not make me smarter than you. I want each of you to make one meaningful contribution to the art of medicine as a whole. One new treatment. One new test. You can do it, because you are better than I am."

Medical students are more knowledgeable now than at any time in history. Every objective measure of student achievement shows an improvement in their quality. Current students in medical school have the same amount of time that their predecessors did—four years—to learn a mountain of information those predecessors never had to learn. I tell them, "You have to learn everything I did in school, *and* you have to learn about everything developed recently."

Even so, the pass rate on the Internal Medicine Boards is 30 points higher than it was in the past, and the average score on the United States Medical Licensing Examination is constantly rising. Newly graduated residents must stay continually current, because recertification is the law of the land every 10 years, whereas those graduating residency 25 years ago had to pass the test only once and never have to prove themselves again. Scores on the boards have risen year after year, so much so that the National Board of Medical Examiners has had to raise the minimum passing score lest the test become too easy.

Beyond their objective knowledge, today's students are also better than their predecessors in the area of patient communications. When I was a student, we had no training in empathy. If bedside manner didn't come to us naturally, we learned it on the fly or not at all. Training in communication, giving bad news, expressing empathy, and trying to take in the whole person is becoming a standard and accepted part of the medical school curriculum. It is an essential part of training because so often in our efforts to provide no false hope, we doctors provide no hope at all. In many patient interviews, I encountered people who had been healed only to go on and suffer from continuing anxiety and depression because of the pain and despair they had experienced.

Medical students must still complete gross anatomy lab and memorize reams of data on biochemistry, but today many schools also go to considerable lengths to try to get students to cultivate and retain sensitivity. This tradition goes back to the father of medical training, the great 19th-century Canadian physician Sir William Osler, who declared, "Medicine is an art, not a trade." My own school is one of many that routinely employs actors as "standardized patients" so that students can practice interviewing patients, giving bad news, and generally being a decent human being.

At SUNY Downstate, where I teach, second-year students are required to take a course called Essentials of Clinical Medicine, which includes students themselves acting as patients with problems ranging from heart disease to erectile dysfunction. More of the year is devoted to sensitivity training and communication (20 percent) than to cardiology (less than 5 percent).

One morning, on the floors at Kings County Hospital Center, the largest municipal hospital in New York City, a student was presenting a case to me. She told me the patient's age, gender, marital status, employment, hobbies, religion, sexual orientation, mood, and status of his relationship with his family and friends. I finally had to interrupt to ask, "What is the patient here for?" The answer: a routine kidney infection. Although I was a little frustrated, I realized that this was an enormous success. The student was following her training to see even a routine patient in terms of his entire life situation. More than at any time in the past, we are training well-rounded physicians; men and women who are truly practicing Osler's art in their attention to patients, body and soul.

It was once considered impossible for humans to break the four-minute mile. Now the top speed is more than 10 seconds less than that. I contend that the same is true in medical education. With years of efforts, I believe that the top-rated students have greatly exceeded their forebears. I think we could expect even greater achievements from them, if they were encouraged.

WE SADDLE MEDICAL students with hundreds of thousands of dollars in student loans; they accept that. We ask them to learn mountains of information; they accept that. We ask them to learn communication and sensitivity in a way never asked of me in school 20 years ago; they accept that, too. Then, when they stagger over the finish line, we basically say, "You haven't seen anything! We were the real thing. You are going to be miserable." No wonder they flee primary care and take refuge in high-paid subspecialties. No wonder that not even 2 percent of physicians choose the physician-scientist road that devotes them to a life of science as well as service. If we want, as I do, to have students who are not only able but *willing* to assault incurable diseases, we need to support and encourage them.

In the fight to see students better regarded and treated more respectfully, I expected the old-guard physicians like Sheldon Landesman to be my enemy and the students to be my allies. But I have heard second-year students argue for an hour about how it was all better in the past. Where did they hear such a thing?

When I approached the Organization of Student Representatives of the Association of American Medical Colleges (AAMC) about distributing a survey on student satisfaction, the student reps rejected it, saying, "This is not an issue of national importance." Think about that: the students themselves believe that it is not an important national issue that today's medical students, the flower of this generation in terms of intelligence and ability, are being systematically demoralized by their teachers.

Henry Sondheimer is the director of the Student Affairs Section of the AAMC, which sets the goals and objectives for training in every school in the country. Henry is warm, sympathetic, and entirely in agreement with me that today's medical students are somehow being poisoned with the narrow-mind virus. Henry says, "It's from faculty who are very negative. They see the amount of clinical work they have to do to support themselves increasing, and the faculty don't like it. So they pass that attitude on to the students. It is older physicians lamenting what they feel is an increased workload on them. The truth is just what you said. There is more great stuff to do for patients all the time, and the education gets better and better, but somehow this doesn't translate into a better feeling about medicine. What we need is a national cheerleader to point this out to them. To get them excited about the great things going on in medicine."

I expected the AAMC leadership to be some evil oligarchy perpetuating old narrow-minded views. It turns out they are just as frustrated as I am by students stuck in this attitude.

The survey I'd proposed to the AAMC's student representatives consisted of two simple questions: Do you feel medicine was better to practice 25 years ago? If so, where did you get this idea? Although that group chose not to respond, I have sent the same survey to all the students I have had in my classes around the country and to all the people who have read my books, and I have asked them to send it to their friends as well. Of the more than 3,000 responses, 80 percent have said that they believe that medicine was better to practice 25 years ago, and 75 percent of those respondents have identified older physicians or teachers as the main source of this opinion. Our students are the best generation, ever, to come out of school, and it is the responsibility of the American Association of Medical Colleges to address the issue that older physicians and faculty are poisoning our next generation of doctors.

It is time for medical school faculty to eschew dogma and look at the facts. It is time for them to become true coaches for their students. It is time for all of us to take healing the minds of medical students as seriously as we take preventing myocardial infarction.

It is not true that medicine was better 25 years ago. In residency 25 years ago, a physician was allowed to work 100 hours a week or more and have the functional capacity of someone legally drunk. Is that what we are proud of? Doctors 25 years ago thought that acid caused ulcers; now we cure ulcers with 10 days of antibiotics. Doctors 25 years ago had more "autonomy," but studies have shown that allowing doctors to use "individual judgment" is worse for patients than requiring them to work in teams. The evidence is that uniform, standard, regimented care plans according to algorithms is better.

It is time to stop teaching medical students to feel sorry for themselves because of managed care and start making them feel that they have the power to do something about it. The health insurance industry is impeding the best scientific minds of our generation and, by extension, the general welfare of millions of Americans. Physicians, who as a group are generally conservative, have been waiting passively for people outside the profession to find a way to insure every American. Instead of complaining about managed care and lack of coverage, physicians need to tackle these issues themselves. They need energy and enthusiasm to defeat this monstrous problem. Young doctors in particular need encouragement from their mentors to do something about it. They don't need to hear about how great it was in the good old days before managed care. They need to hear that managed care is a problem and that they, as the best and brightest, can and should take a lead role in helping government and society solve it.

A chorus of narrow-minded voices is drowning out the good news that doctors today are able to cure more diseases, heal more people, and relieve more suffering than ever before in human history. The popular press is packed with works describing our failures, our weaknesses, and a method of drug development that is so often illogical and unproductive that it would not take a paranoid person much to envision conspiracy. If you go to a bookstore and look at the medical section, you will find many works on how doctors and pharmaceutical companies are geared more toward making profits than toward finding new, meaningful therapies.

It is not that such voices are wrong. I simply seek to bring some balance to the discussion. The medical profession faces difficult challenges both in curing life-threatening illnesses and in helping solve the nation's health insurance crisis. My hope is that a crescendo of understanding of how far we've come will deafen students to their teachers' discouraging words. My hope is that this volume will open young minds to the idea that it is possible to beat heart disease, stroke, cancer, and all disease that plagues humanity. This book covers, in a purposely euphoric manner, medical advances that would once have been called miracles but are now merely routine. My interviews with physicians and patients have yielded stories of hope and optimism and triumph. This is the best time ever to come out of medical school and training. And that is a fact to inspire and uplift not only students, residents, and young doctors but all of us who must, at some point in our lives, rely on the art of medicine to see us through.

CHAPTER 2

A Vocation to Satisfy the Soul

I AM AN INFECTIOUS diseases doctor. I have been taking care of HIV-positive patients for 20 years. I first heard about HIV while in college in 1982; I was 19 years old, working as a teaching assistant for physiology professor Dr. Phillip Stein. He was an enormous character, a classroom performer who told completely unfunny jokes with such good humor that we laughed just to make him happy.

"They say it will achieve bubonic plague proportions," he said one day in his office.

"What will?" I asked.

"AIDS," he said. "I just got back from a meeting. It's all they are talking about."

I was typing up his class notes and doing research on thyroid glands for a reason I cannot remember, but even then I knew I had to go to medical school. Looking back, I now understand that the word *calling* means something you simply must do, for reasons you cannot name.

My major concerns were getting the grades I needed to get into medical school and finishing college in three years; the latter because I knew everything else would be long. I had rarely been in a hospital. No one in my family was sick. No one had an incurable disease that I felt driven to cure or treat. But I was in a mad rush to become a doctor.

I want to change the world. I want to make a difference. I rehearsed statements like that in a mirror while preparing for medical school interviews. It would take at least another ten years before I stumbled on the reason for my calling.

I graduated with distinction from the State University of New York at New Paltz. I had the honor of being named "Outstanding Senior" in two departments. I was very proud to have this honor, a rare achievement. Yet I also felt sorry for myself: I was on the waiting list at two medical schools but had received no acceptances.

My father was a New York City police captain, by way of law school, nursing school, and finally a degree in economics. He said that he would help me, that he "had it all arranged."

I was stunned. My father was a difficult man. When my mother wanted to teach my brothers and me the language of her parents, he'd blocked it, saying, "We're in America now. If that country was so great, why did they leave? Read Shakespeare."

I had not exactly gotten encouragement from my father when I told him I wanted to be a doctor.

"What the hell do you want to do that for?" he said. "Doctors are nothing but specialized mechanics."

This really helped my drive. One thing I can say about my father was that he taught me never to be dissuaded from my goals, often by strengthening my resolve to oppose him.

But here I was, hearing my father say, "The dean of admissions at a certain medical school recently got into trouble. Your father"—he loved referring to himself in the third person—"was in a position to do this person a favor and extricate him from his difficulty. He owes me a favor."

Huh? All of a sudden I felt I had entered a movie. "What do you mean?" I asked.

"Your father has arranged it for you to get a position in medical school. I have put in the fix for you."

I was furious. "I won't go. If I can't get in on my own steam, I won't go." My father was in enormously good physical shape. Telling him no was a scary thing.

"What? Your father is offering you a favor and you turn him down? I am expecting the call within the hour to confirm it."

Now I knew what movie I was in—*The Godfather.*

"You are spitting in my face," he continued. "This is what love means. Your father is taking care of you."

My father was, and is, one of the least compassionate, least sympathetic people I have ever known. When my heart is bleeding about some issue, such as HIV, he'll say, "It's a form of population control, kid."

I remained adamant. "I won't go," I said. I didn't want to owe my father a favor, and I didn't want to achieve my calling in this way. My father had worked for years with the Mafia in Brooklyn — on the police side, I believe.

My father softened from scary man to intellectual cop who read three books a week and quoted Shakespeare at meals.

Despite being completely unsympathetic in his rhetoric, he did have something about him that taught me to protect people. Hospitals were started as houses of "hospitality" for spiritual pilgrims along the path from Europe to the Middle East. The Knights Hospitallers were crusaders who changed their ways and took seriously the commandment "Do not kill." They set up hospitals to protect the weak and the innocent. It took me years as a doctor to feel empathy, to undergo suffering with someone. But I could always defend people. I could protect them. To this day, as a doctor I can easily relate to the concept of protection, whereas empathy is something I have to work at.

I once asked my patients, most of whom have followed me through five different jobs and locations in the 17 years since I finished my residency, why they tolerate some of my behavior. I am late. I interrupt them midsentence. I am hyper.

They respond: "Because when we are sick, we know you will do anything you have to, to protect us. If someone is doing something wrong, you will get mad at them and yell at them. When you get mad for us, we relax and know we are protected."

My father has no verbal ability to express empathy, yet he does have a wish to protect people and do favors. So, I suppose, love is an action.

THE FOLLOWING DAY was the Friday before Memorial Day weekend, a week after I graduated as a highly qualified unemployed person with no future.

My father said, "I've made an arrangement. On Tuesday we'll go to the Polish embassy. I'm a member of the organization of Polish cops and firemen, and we'll meet the Polish ambassador on Tuesday, and you'll apply to medical school in Poland."

"What are you talking about? We're not Polish!"

"Don't interrupt me! You now have a Polish grandmother."

Three days later, organized over a holiday weekend, I was having a vodka in the Polish embassy in New York.

The head of the Polish Organization said, "He looks like an intelligent boy."

Forty-eight hours after that I was in Warsaw. The following day, I was living in Krakow. Poland was then a Communist state, but at least martial law was over. I plunged into Polish language courses. I acclimatized. I applied to Polish medical school, and the Polish government, starved for U.S. dollars, accepted me to seven schools with one application. I relaxed a little. I met Polish girls, and the first Polish word I learned was the word for beer. Girls and beer. But not always in that order. I relaxed a lot.

In fact, I was willing to go to any lengths to achieve my calling. I left the States in a heartbeat. I got into medical school on my own steam. I earned it.

Two months later, at the end of summer, I got an excited call from New York. My brother and father told me: "Hey, Con, guess what?

You just got into two schools in New York! The only thing is, you have to get back in thirty-six hours to sign up in person or you lose the spot."

Flights in Communist Poland were disorganized. *Terrific,* I thought. *I get into a U.S. medical school, but I am going to lose the spot because I can't get out of the country.* On a midnight train to Warsaw, I felt like I was escaping prison. I arrived at medical school the day before classes started.

FAST-FORWARD TO MY last year of residency. I didn't know what to specialize in. I was leaning toward oncology, with the goal of doing bone marrow transplants. My main teacher at the time was the director of critical care, David. I love him. Every time someone called him "Doctor," he'd say, "David, please!" He sometimes made seemingly insensitive statements : "Why are we rounding on all these dead people? Don't we have any live patients here? Get a consult from the Hemlock Society for this patient."

David was a beautiful guy. Blond hair, trained in California, like a beach bum with brains. Always cool and relaxed, except when it came to patient care. It turned out that the blond-haired California boy was 100 percent maniacal about having things done perfectly for patients. And when patients were dying, which was every day, this seemingly cynical wiseass took time out to meet with families.

It was 1991. The AIDS epidemic seemed to be reaching bubonic plague proportions. We were in the hospital adjacent to Lincoln Center for the Performing Arts in Manhattan, confronting death. Confronting HIV at a time when there was, essentially, a 100 percent death rate. We had only a few medications, all of them ineffective.

Every day, the most talented and accomplished people of our culture were being brought in. The opera singer with dementia. The landscape artist gone blind. The trombone player with Kaposi's sarcoma on his lip. I sometimes thought that HIV was intent on destroying in patients precisely the thing they loved most.

There was David. He sat for an hour with patients and their loved ones, explaining everything. "For I have understood the large hearts of heroes," says Walt Whitman. David, my hero, never flinched.

When it came time for me to finish my residency, I didn't know what to do with myself. David said, "I have a part-time job in the little hospital down the street, St. Clare's. Half the beds of the hospital are for AIDS patients. You can work for me for a year while you decide. I will be there ten hours a week, and you can run things when I'm not there. See patients. Run morning report"—the main teaching exercise for a hospital—"and organize things."

MY PROGRAM DIRECTOR was a Harvard-trained gastroenterologist and the picture of academic achievement. The year before, he had given me a three-day suspension for insubordination. The problem was that, instead of simply following orders, I had continually asked the faculty and my supervising residents to explain the reasons for those orders.

They would say "Conrad, get a CBC [complete blood count] on that patient."

"Why?"

"Because we want to document it."

"*Why?*"

"Because we want to put it in the chart."

"*Why?* What are you going to *do* with the information?"

"Get it because I am telling you to, that's why!"

"In that case, since you can't tell my why you want it or what you are going to do with it, then get it yourself."

Twenty minutes later I am summoned to the program director's office. "Conrad, if you are going to learn *one thing* this year, you are going to learn respect for authority. If I hear of *one* more act of insubordination, you are going to be suspended from this program." I respond, "I want to be chief resident." "Are you crazy?" he says. "I barely mentioned this to the faculty, and some of them said they would resign if you were made chief resident." Some time passes, and an attending faculty member tells me to stick a needle in a patient for some unknown reason. "Why?" I ask. In about three nanoseconds, I am in the program director's office "You are *out of here*! I told you I was going to teach you respect for authority. Now get the hell out of here! You are suspended for three days."

"Why?" I ask.

The academic gastroenterologist spits out his response: "You are a philosophical guy, Conrad. Go sit on a mountain for three days and think about it!" I wonder if he regrets there is no corporal punishment system in medical education. He looks like he wants to hit me.

A year passes. I become a senior resident. I continue to ask my "whys," in a more muted fashion, but insist the residents and students ask me "Why?" about everything I am doing. In fact, I get angry if they don't. "Are you a waiter?" I ask. "Why are you doing that test? What are you going to do with the information?"

At the end of that year, the program director had written in my evaluation: "It is good to finally see one resident who has the respect of his troops."

Around this time I was summoned to the chairman's office. *Uh-oh! What did I do now?* I thought as I ran through the list of all the many people I may have pissed off.

The chairman was Gerald Turino, a full Columbia University professor and a titan in the American Thoracic Society. He was charged with making St. Luke's-Roosevelt Hospital an academic powerhouse. He had helped develop the first intracardiac pressure monitoring tubes and was as big as they come in academic medicine.

"We want you to be chief resident," Dr. Turino told me. "You have a year off between residency and the chief year. Make it useful. Congratulations!"

Following that meeting, I went to see my program director. He was smiling a big smile. "Congratulations!" he said.

"I don't understand," I said. "Last year you said I was insubordinate."

The program director replied, "That was last year, when you were a junior. Now we call it 'leadership.'"

A short time later, the program director and I were discussing my plan to accept David's offer to spend a year at the tiny St. Clare's Hospital. It was so small that most physicians in New York, even a few blocks away, did not know it was there. But I loved my teacher, and I wanted to go. At the time, I thought it was a whim. Now I know that a calling can bring you to strange places.

The program director was clear: "Don't go to St. Clare's. Once you have a 'nowhere' place like St. Clare's on your CV, your career in academic medicine is over. No one will want you."

I realized that he really cared about me and was giving me his best advice.

"In terms of your career, it would be better for you to take a year off and travel," he said. He was sincere. He meant well.

I went to St. Clare's.

DURING THE YEAR at St. Clare's, I built classrooms and took care of HIV patients day and night.

One day, an intern who had been assisting in some course for medical education walked up to me and said, "You are a pretty good teacher. They are expanding some courses for the USMLE [United States Medical Licensing Examination], and maybe you want to teach in them."

"Sure," I answered. "Why not?"

I picked up the phone, and on a whim I started teaching.

Also during my year at St. Clare's, a woman I had been seeing for two years, Cristina, a beautiful French-Italian MD-PhD who could curse at me in three languages, says: "Do you want to marry me?"

"No, I am not ready," I told her.

Cristina was the orchid of my life. Delicate. Refined. Generous and extremely tolerant. At least until now.

"In that case, lose my phone number. I don't want to see you anymore."

Two weeks later, I was out of my mind with longing for her. I called her and said, "I have changed my mind. I love you and want to marry you!"

"Too late! You only want me now because you can't have me. Because you are a pushy American man. I was never important to you, never a priority for you. I am tired of crying in a bathroom over you. *Ça suffit, tu es fou! C'est fini!*"

I sent flowers every day for a month, along with poems and letters with generous amounts of begging, all to no effect. Her words rang in my ears: *I was never important to you, never a priority.* I made a decision. Cristina was going into infectious diseases at one of the best programs in the country. I decided to show her that she was a priority to me by applying to the same specialty. I decide to go to the same program. A year before, I had asked her about her choice and my own indecision. She said: "Infectious diseases is not for loud American men. It is for delicate European women." I did not get the girl, but I am, today, a specialist in infectious diseases because of the best reason in the world.

Love.

By the end of the whole application and acceptance process, it became clear that my attempt to show my devotion was a failure.

"Ahhh! You've ruined my life! That fellowship was the only thing I was looking forward to, and you've ruined it," Cristina said.

"I want to marry you," I said.

"Well, they haven't called a phyciatric consultant on me. Well, I haven't been declared incompetent," she replied, "so I don't see any reason I should marry you."

In a rare moment of good judgment, I decided to be a man and withdraw from the program. I had been accepted to other programs as well, but they wouldn't take me unless I had a clean release from the infectious diseases program. I told the program director some of the story and asked to be released.

He said, "No, I don't release people from professional obligations for personal reasons."

I was stuck. I made the best of it and prepared to do the fellowship.

In the meantime, I returned to my original hospital, where I had completed my residency, to do my year as the chief resident. A month into it, David, my favorite teacher and the critical care director, asked me to cover for him as the attending physician in the intensive care unit because he was going to be out sick for a while.

I agreed and started to work. A few weeks went by, but David did not return. I made calls and finally got a message back: "David is hospitalized and he has given a very clear instruction. No one is to visit. No one is to call. No one is to write. He specifically orders everyone to leave him alone."

Twenty minutes later, of course, I was across town entering his hospital room. Weak, lying in bed completely wasted, he looked like a concentration camp victim, a ghost. In an instant I could see he had AIDS.

He got mad at me. "Can't you follow a simple three-part instruction? I told you not to come!"

I started crying. I knew what would happen. "I couldn't stay away." Overcome with the emotion of seeing him devastated, I blurted out, "I love you, you know!" Then I tried to smile. "Besides that, you know I can't follow instructions."

We spent a few minutes together before I yielded to his intense need for privacy. I hadn't realized it before, but David was a very, very, very private man. He and his lover both had AIDS. Doth died in a few months.

I returned to St. Clare's and finished out my chief year. I covered the rest of David's months as the ICU attending physician, and I gave the eulogy at his memorial.

My teacher was dead of AIDS. At the end of the year, I moved across town to begin my fellowship.

WHEN SIR WILLIAM OSLER, the father of modern medicine, wrote, "Happiness lies in the absorption in some vocation which satisfies the soul," he could well have been writing about my two years of fellowship.

Memorial Sloan-Kettering Cancer Center is one of the most exalted and beautifully run places in the whole world. Packed with money and donations, it is a magnet for the top 1 percent of minds and ability from everywhere.

I never quite felt at home there because I always felt I arrived under false pretenses. Every day I worked with world leaders. Nobel Prize winners gave noon conferences. The head of the U.S. Centers for Disease Control and Prevention stopped by. The head of tuberculosis control for the World Health Organization taught on tuberculosis. Dr. John Bartlett, one of the most important authors in the Western world on the intestinal organism *Clostridium difficile,* gave a noon conference.

I did not know that Dr. Bartlett was the head of the Infectious Diseases Department at Johns Hopkins Hospital. After the conference, I exclaimed, "Wow! You described *that!*" I asked, "Gosh, you described a new organism! That's so cool! How come you didn't name it after your girlfriend or your wife?"

Dr. Bartlett smiled and said, "I thought of that, but since it causes severe diarrhea, my wife asked me where the bug was found, so I decided against it."

He smiled and I thought he was nice. The rest of the fellows and attending physicians shifted in their seats. Eyes rolled.

In the department one day, I looked at a plaque on the wall. It was the patent for aerosolized pentamidine, at the time a main prophylactic medication for the most common opportunistic infection in AIDS. "Why is that there?" I asked.

"Because we invented it," said the others, looking at me like I had not gotten enough oxygen at birth.

I consulted on cancer patients who were being taken care of by people whose names seemed vaguely familiar.

"Why do I know that name?" I once asked about the lymphoma attending physician.

"Because she wrote the chapter on lymphoma in *Harrison's Principles of Internal Medicine*," came the reply. *Harrison's Principles of Internal Medicine* has been the leading textbook of medicine for the last half century. Again, the same look.

Memorial Sloan-Kettering has the most rarified and beautiful atmosphere of science and scholarship I have ever seen. It consists of a nearly eight-block compound connected by tunnels to the Rockefeller University, a hatchery for Nobel Prizes, and Cornell Medical Center. A tunnel connects the fellows' residency building to the hospital. You can be there for your entire life and never set foot outside the hospital or the laboratory. It is like the vitreous chamber of the inner eye, an immunologically privileged area. When Sir William Osler, the father of modern medicine wrote, "Happiness lies in the absorption in some vocation which satisfies the soul," this is what he meant.

The center was founded in the 1940s by the same men who ran General Motors. Throughout the 1930s, they had mastered the concept of individual teams for research and development in the automotive industry. A team on the engine, a team on the brakes, one on the transmission. Alfred P. Sloan was the chairman of General Motors. One day his head of research and development, Charles F. Kettering, said to Sloan something like "Hey, we have done so well on cars, why don't we cure cancer?" and that is how it started.

The chief of the Infectious Diseases Service was Dr. Donald Armstrong. He had been there for 40 years, originally as the chief resident. The first patient to die of AIDS in New York City was under his care. He was the president of the Infectious Diseases Society of America and was, to me, like a combination of the Statue of Liberty and Ray Charles in terms of stature.

I tried for two years to get him to laugh. One day, on rounds I asked this grim bastion about his history at Sloan-Kettering. This was not too intelligent on my part. Don Armstrong was in the business of taking care of patients, developing new drugs, and trying to cure disease. He trained dozens of department chairs and division heads. A "Donald Armstrong product" was the peak of academic-clinical-scientific excellence. He was not thrilled with a Mr. Personality type like me.

Even so, one day on rounds, I asked about his history at Sloan-Kettering in my own inimitable way. "Gee, what did you do here in the 1960s?" I said. "There was no HIV, no MRIs, no CT scans, no carbapenem antibiotics, no cephalosporins. What exactly did you do all day?"

It sounds immensely stupid right now, but at the time I actually wanted to know what fellows in infectious diseases had done in the days when 90 percent of what we have now to offer patients did not exist. It seemed to me that all they could have done was watch people die. (I remember my father once asking me at the time, "So, kid, how's it going in the world's best-documented abattoir? Still keeping the trouble makers sedated?" I didn't know then that *abattoir* was just a five-dollar word for "slaughterhouse," but I didn't like the tone of the question.)

"We worked hard and took care of our patients. That's what we did," Dr. Armstrong said in a tone of voice that made me think I should place myself on the organ donor list. Then something strange happened: he went on. "When I came here, my friends were going to NASA to put a man on the moon or go to the bottom of the sea to explore. I came here to eradicate cancer."

This statement has stayed with me ever since. It is part of the reason I have written this book. The sense of "I am in medicine to eradicate disease" has been lost in the profession. Students in school and residents in training compete now for high-paying subspecialties to hide from dealing with the biggest killers. In the 1960s, when physicians could not actually do much, they kept hope alive with the thought that they were always on the verge of the cure. Today, that hope seems to have died. In it's place is fear. It was the most exciting thing for me about this environment, a complete commitment, a full immersion, and a devotion to medicine.

AFTER TWO YEARS of fellowship at Sloan-Kettering, I looked for my career path. I asked the head of the basic science HIV laboratory to let me come in. He said no. "You are too uncoordinated, Conrad. Can you really see yourself handling live HIV virus in a lab? I can't do it. You will kill yourself or someone else."

I was angry and frustrated. What would I do? I knew by then that AIDS would be the plague of our time. It was 1994, and the epidemic was exploding. There were four approved medications, none of which controlled the disease. I desperately wanted to be in the game. I felt my calling again.

By accident, I found out that an anonymous serosurvey was being done of all new babies born in New York State. A heel stick was being used to collect data on the rate of HIV infection in newborns. But there was something sad and strange going on. If a baby tested positive, the information was not passed on to the mother unless she had specifically asked for the test to be done. It seemed criminal to me not to inform mothers that their babies were going to get sick and, moreover, that they themselves would, too. But at the time, there was no truly effective therapy for AIDS. There was also the enormous issue of patient confidentiality: no test was supposed to be administered without explicit written consent of the adult.

Later that year, a landmark study of anti-HIV medications in mothers was published showing that when azidothymidine (AZT, now called zidovudine) was given to the mother, the rate of HIV transmission from mother to child decreased from 25 percent to 8 percent. This was explosive news: for the first time ever, it showed clearly and unequivocally that HIV medications could prevent death. The study was stopped once it became clear that it was unethical to continue the placebo arm of the trial. All HIV-positive mothers were then given AZT, and that is the way it has been ever since.

My life was about to change completely.

I had been on some committees in some physician groups as a resident. I was already an experienced lobbyist and had been to Albany and to Washington, D.C., a few times to argue for funding for education on issues related to HIV. At the time, I was vociferously on the side of the AIDS activists, the clear underdogs. They were passionate and sincere, even if they were socially inappropriate, over the top. I fit right in.

At a meeting of the state medical society, I heard about a woman named Nettie Mayersohn, a member of the New York State Assembly from Queens who was trying to pass legislation that would make it mandatory for hospitals to offer HIV testing to all pregnant women. Prior to this legislative attempt, Nettie was classified as a left-leaning feminist.

Once a law passes in a big state like New York, it is often adopted in other states. All Nettie wanted was to give pregnant women the opportunity to find out their HIV status so that those who tested positive could take AZT to prevent transmission of the virus to their babies. Her proposal also allowed for treatment of the babies, in the event that AZT failed, and would thus help prevent opportunistic infections.

What mother would not want to know if her baby was sick? I thought. *What is the big deal?* However, Nettie's position was enormously unpopular with activists, who misconstrued her call for mandatory (or automatic) *offering* of HIV testing as a call for mandatory testing. They did not understand that her proposal to require hospitals to make the offer left women free to accept or decline that offer. They absolutely hated the idea of testing in this way. "Automatic offering," in their minds, was instantly translated into "mandatory without consent." Overnight, she was reclassified as an ultra-right-wing invader of privacy, a counterrevolutionary.

Many of the people I had sided with before visited the state capital in 10-to-1 ratios against the testing. My first child had recently been born, so the activists' stance was bizarre to me. I understand now that they were looking at the privacy aspect of HIV status.

I wrote a piece on health care policy and law concerning HIV, babies, and mothers. Ordinarily, I found writing research articles to be excruciating. Day and night for over a year, I had been collecting hundreds of pages of data on fungus in the blood of cancer patients. It was torture. I never published those findings. But my piece on "baby AIDS," as the issue became known, flew out of my hands in an hour. AIDS had become a high-profile disease. Under the Clinton administration, funding for research began to pour in. Pharmaceutical manufacturers began to invest billions. Yet, for patients who were young, vital, and politically aware, progress was still way too slow. People began to wear red ribbons. Celebrities became activists.

Strange and unique things began to happen at national scientific meetings. Clinicians and researchers presented their data to their colleagues. But now activists showed up, too. I recalled one meeting at which a group of activists walked in, one by one, and crossed the stage carrying large white cards with single letters. What's going on? On a beat, like a cue in a Broadway play, they formed a line so that the letters spelled out "HURRY UP!" I knew then that they were members of the AIDS Coalition to Unleash Power. They flipped the cards to spell out "ACT UP!" and shouted the words aloud.

Cool! I thought. The audience of clinician-scientists was frozen in their seats. What next? Two people ran up and threw buckets of what looked like blood on the presenting scientist. The presenter, covered in what was turned out to be strawberry syrup, started to cry. The ACT UP members screamed, "This is the blood of the people who are dying while you are taking your time talking!" They marched out chanting, "Act up!"

Normally the U.S. Food and Drug Administration takes 10 years between the submission of data and the final approval of medications.

The first protease inhibitor, indinavir, was approved in 42 days. Indinavir is lifesaving when combined with other HIV medications.

BACK AT SLOAN-KETTERING, Donald Armstrong did not like the AIDS ribbon I wore, which puzzled me.

He did not tell me to take it off. It would probably have been a sign of weakness to him if I did, because Armstrong was a fierce individualist. When he asked for test results, like an X-ray, he would say, "Did you see it yourself?" When a biopsy came out, he would say, "Did you look at the biopsy through the microscope yourself?" One day he'd asked what a particular attending physician, a huge authority in his area, had recommended for a patient. I told him, but I also said that I didn't agree with the plan. I expected him to suspend me for insubordination. Instead he asked, "Are you sure you are right?"

"Yes."

"Did you tell him to go to hell?"

"No, but I didn't follow his recommendation."

Case closed. Dr. Armstrong never said "Good work," not in this instance or in any other. He just moved on to the next case. Good work was its own reward.

It didn't make sense to me that Dr. Armstrong didn't like the red AIDS ribbons. Here was a man who took poor, uninsured AIDS patients into a large private institution. He took care of them one on one, at a time when no one knew whether you could get HIV from casual contact. He bucked the administration of a cancer center that wondered what he was doing with HIV in cases without cancer. He put his job on the line for them.

When I finally asked about his obvious distaste for the AIDS ribbon, he said, "I don't like dividing patients into groups. We take care of everybody here. We don't make exceptions. That thing you wear means that group gets extra attention. Everyone here gets the attention they need."

I thought about this for a while—partly because I did not want to look like I was knuckling under, and partly because I thought he might be wrong. Didn't AIDS need extra attention? "Dr. Armstrong," I asked, "doesn't it make you sad when these young people die?"

"It makes me sad when old people die, too," he said.

I took off the ribbon.

IT CAME TIME for me to finish my fellowship and look for a job. In a leadership training house like Sloan-Kettering, you do not walk off into just any job. You are expected to go into research and work at a medical school or an academic community hospital. That year, however, there was only one spot in New York at a university program, and I was not even in the running. The two other graduating fellows were, and one of them got it. I, on the other hand, had another type of awakening.

Don Armstrong called me into his office. When I sat down, he told me the faculty had decided it would let me sit for the boards.

"What do you mean 'let me'?" I asked. "Was there ever any doubt?"

"Well, Conrad, at the faculty meeting we came to the conclusion that you are the least knowledgeable fellow ever to go through this training program. However, there was consensus that you are a generally nice guy and that, hopefully, you will study for your boards and pass."

I was stunned. I had been teaching all over for three years, and I was the lead author on my first textbook. I had also won my first Teacher of the Year Award in a national venue. So, with a steady diet of feeling pretty smart, it was very hard to comprehend Dr. Armstrong's evaluation. I would have understood it if the faculty had not liked my personality, but I had never been called ignorant before.

"And what exactly is the basis for the faculty's judgment about my knowledge?" I asked.

"Well, Conrad," he said, "when we are in conference, do you see any other fellows asking questions? When we are on rounds, do you hear anyone else asking the kinds of things you ask about?"

Wow! I thought. *No job and I am dumb, too! Well, it can only get better.*

A few weeks before the end of my fellowship, I heard in passing from an old acquaintance that a community-based program, the Community Family Planning Council, was looking for someone to do HIV work. I was interviewed the next day, then hired the day after that to be the medical director of the council's HIV program in a Brooklyn neighborhood that I'd never heard of before. That neighborhood, East New York, was a notch below Crown Heights and Bedford-Stuyvesant in terms of safety and was classified as an "underserved" area.

At the graduation party for the fellows in my class, people took turns announcing their new positions. When I said where I was going, the party looked like a meeting of the Facial Paralysis Support Group. No one moved.

Regardless of what anyone else thought, when I began my new job, a funny thing happened: I started to feel happy. The Community Family Planning Council was one of ten citywide clinics that were remnants of President Lyndon Johnson's War on Poverty, and many of my coworkers were living as if it were still the 1960s. At staff meetings, people held hands and sang "We Shall Overcome." I worked one day a week on the mobile van outside the Lower East Side needle exchange. The rest of the time, I worked as the lead physician in a remoter than remote health center now named after Betty Shabazz, Malcolm X's wife. I saw patients, set policy for HIV care, and did quality assurance throughout the organization. I was suddenly the highest medical authority in the building. For the first time in my professional life, I felt indispensable. If I didn't fix a problem, no one else besides me would do it, because there was no one else. Many of the patients I have now, in 2009, are people I met in my first month or two out of training in 1994.

THAT YEAR, THE "baby AIDS" issue heated up. Nettie Mayersohn started her legislative push. I called Mayersohn's office to volunteer to speak on behalf of passing the bill regarding HIV testing for pregnant women. It was my first formal testimony in front of a legislative body. The activists were out in force against the bill. The Satan of the moment was Mayersohn, who a year or two before had been declared Woman of the Year by the National Organization for Women. I met her for the first time as I entered the council chambers at city hall.

"Well, hello, darling, how are you? Thanks for coming," she said.

At five feet tall, on a hot day, she made me think of a Jewish leprechaun. From that moment on, she felt like a mother to me. I would not have been surprised if she pulled out milk and cookies.

She said, "Don't worry too much. Just make your point, and we will fight the big fight in the capital next month."

Mayersohn always knew something that often escapes me: when to fight all the way, and when to make your point and leave. Over the course of the next six months, I went with her to give testimony throughout the state, including legislative office visits in the capital.

We doctors are not paid lobbyists, which tends to make legislators pay more attention to us. But all the other doctors here were "socially appropriate"—that is, reasonable, intelligent, and mature—no match for the activist circus; the ranting lunatics who threw strawberry syrup at people. And then there was me. I loved my screaming matches with the activists who painted the bill as a bite out of civil rights.

I was surprised to have found my niche, but I was surprised still more by the fact that Mayersohn's bill passed. The law of the land in New York State became the mandatory offer of HIV testing to all pregnant women. Once the law was in place, far less than 1 percent of women refused to be tested. Overnight, pediatric HIV virtually ceased to exist in New York State. The rule was soon adopted in other states as well, and the number of children born HIV-positive plummeted from 2,000 a year to under 200. With new medications, the transmission rate from mother to child fell to less than 2 percent, and for those fully compliant with medications, the rate fell to less than 1 percent. That means that, today, virtually every child born in the United States to an HIV-positive mother will be healthy—as long as we are testing the mother and offering her the medications during pregnancy.

I cannot say that my medical practice has been unique. I cannot claim to write a prescription with such panache that HIV leaps back inside a T cell and hides forever. I can be sure, however, that I was instrumental in passing this law with the great Nettie Mayersohn. I have sometimes wondered whether I was sure I had saved someone's life. It is hard to be sure. Most of the fatal illnesses I have prevented were not with the result of a prescription, a procedure, or a device; rather, they were the result of my helping to pass a law, one that has led to the virtual elimination of children with AIDS in the United States. Those parts of my personality that made me too large, too loud, too clumsy to get into a lab made me just right to join the fight against AIDS. The same irritation and impatience that made me hate writing up research data facilitated the writing I did to help pass Mayersohn's law. The point of this story is to consider that if you are working hard, learning, and trying to do the right thing but still not succeeding, the solution may not be changing how you do your work. It may be changing *where* you do it and what you are working on.

A few years after Nellie Mayersohn's HIV testing legislation passed, the subject of partner notification in HIV came up. If a person is found to be HIV-positive, should it be mandatory to inform his or her sexual and/or needle-sharing contacts that they are at risk? I had several patients, almost all women, who'd become infected with HIV after heterosexual contact with men who did not inform them of their HIV status. Again, Nettie Mayersohn rode in with legislation. Again, legions of civil libertarians and activists protested, insisting that mandatory notification was a violation of an HIV-positive person's privacy. Again I asked, "What about the rights of the uninfected person to be protected?" History repeated itself, and the bill passed.

One difference this time was that, as a result of the previous legislative effort, the governor had appointed me to the New York State AIDS

Advisory Council, a body of clinicians, activists, public health officials, and finance people designated to advise the legislature on policy issues concerning HIV. Now my yelling was legitimized. This took a little of the fun out of it. Still, I felt fully alive at these times of conflict, because I knew that my calling had sent me in this direction.

OVER TIME, I became increasingly frustrated with the inefficiency of the system in place at the Community Family Planning Council. I started to drive people crazy by being too pushy: *Why isn't this fixed? What the hell is wrong here?*

By chance, one day I attended a meeting in our administrative office with the medical director of the HIV program at Bellevue Hospital Center of New York University. We hit it off immediately. Before long, I had a faculty appointment at New York University and was working part-time at Bellevue! Then, after mentioning my teaching experience, I became the morning report teacher at the University Hospital of NYU.

Another chance meeting at NYU, and I heard they needed a program director for one of the large hospitals in Brooklyn. This was a big academic promotion in terms of responsibility. However, it meant leaving the big medical school at NYU. I heard my calling: "Go where the world needs you most." I left, and my patients came with me. Two years later, it was fixed. I then turned to another program that was slated to be shut down. Two years later, that one was fixed as well.

Several years after finishing training, I heard about the fellow from my graduating class who got the only academic position in New York. By this time, I'd had two faculty appointments and was doing what I was meant to do. But apparently my classmate, feeling exploited as the low man on the totem pole, left academics altogether for private practice in a Connecticut suburb.

I was in the emergency department one day seeing patients and teaching. The resident there said, "Wow, Dr. Fischer, you're like a really smart guy! You are like a cesspool of information. You should go on one of those TV game shows and win a million dollars."

"You know what I would do if I won a million dollars?" I replied. "I would be here with you, right now, doing exactly what we are doing."

My ability to respond in such a way helped me to know that I am living my calling—although, thinking back on it, as a 19-year-old medical school applicant, I could not have told you why I felt called.

TEN YEARS AFTER the chance suggestion that I take up teaching USMLE at St. Clare's (the hospital that I was told had "no academic future"), I became the most prolific teacher of medicine in the country. Fifteen years later, I became the world's most prolific author of medical textbooks for the USMLE, students, and residents. I also became known as a person to be brought in as a fixer for training programs on probation or slated to be closed. All based on doing what I loved most in the world.

I was asked to be program director at several places and ultimately became the associate chief of medicine for education at SUNY Downstate Medical Center in Brooklyn. (This came about by chance. Dr. Edmund Bourke, chairman at Downstate, was sitting near me at a national program directors' meeting. Deciding to play on the similarity of his name to that of the 18th-century Irish statesman Edmund Burke, I leaned forward and said, "Do you know what you said two hundred years ago? 'All that is necessary for the triumph of evil is for good men to do nothing.'" Although I quoted Burke as part of a joke, these are in fact words I have chosen to live by.)

When I first came to Downstate, I, like anybody else, wanted to do well and to be effective with the trainees. One day I noticed among the students a rather sullen, withdrawn guy in the corner. I finally asked him, Claudiu, what his story was.

In front of the whole room, he said, "Well, basically, Dr. Fischer, I don't like you. I don't trust you, and I don't know what you are trying to prove here. Actually, not only do I not trust you, I don't even trust people who are like you, and I don't like people who are even like you."

I tried to recall whether I'd worn clean underwear to work that day, because I definitely felt stripped almost naked at that moment. It was such an unexpected answer that I could only smile and make a mental note to never again ask questions I don't want answers to. I also thought that Claudiu must be two steps up the evolutionary ladder from wherever *Homo sapiens* are. As the associate chief of medicine, I may not have had the power over much territory, but I definitely had enormous power to control this young man's chance at promotion. And the entryway into highly sought-after subspecialty fellowships is fragile and almost whimsical. One bad word from an important person, and you are toast. This student took his entire career in his hands by criticizing me, his boss, in public. I found it either the craziest thing I had heard all year, or the most admirable.

That evening on the way out of the building, I was taking the elevator down, and I started chatting with an intern who was not at the morning conference: "How is it going?"

"Great," she said.

"Wow! Why so great?" I asked.

"Because my resident is wonderful. He is a great teacher."

"Who is that?"

"Claudiu."

Small world, I thought.

Soon afterward I bumped into another student on the way to the subway. "How is it going? How's the teaching?"

"Great," came the response. A look of excitement and engagement washed over the student's face.

"What's the best thing that's happening?" I asked.

"My resident is great. He really takes care of us."

"Who is that?"

"Claudiu."

Neither the intern nor the student had been present at the morning's class where Claudiu had eviscerated me. The next morning I entered the hospital with a letter in my hand. It was for Claudiu. The students and I sat down for our usual morning conference. I was struck by the fact that Claudiu made no attempt to contact me at all. No apology. I handed Claudiu the letter. "Open it," I instructed. I half expected him to throw it in my face, but instead I saw in him the first look of fear.

He read the letter to himself and froze. I told myself I should not be enjoying this moment so much. The other residents were aquiver with anticipation.

He then read it aloud for them. What I had given him was a letter of recommendation: "Dear program director, I am writing in support of Claudiu . . . He is . . . excellent . . . honest . . . strong . . . capable . . . And most of all, Claudiu has enormous courage of the type that qualify him for a position of leadership in the future. I heartily recommend him for the fellowship of his choice."

I said, "When you are ready, tell me what you want to specialize in, and we will get that position for you."

Claudiu sat as if paralyzed. The rest of the residents cheered.

That moment set the tone thereafter for the relationship between me and the trainees. I had made it clear that the difference between training in the military or other organizations and training in medicine is that in the latter no one is automatically right because of a position. In medicine, whoever is right, is right. We judge people's statements according to facts, according to our common care for our patients, not rank. I had made it clear to the students that Claudiu's dislike for me was not what mattered. It was not his management of the people who above him that mattered. His treatment of those below him, his ability as a teacher, and his knowledge as a physician were what mattered. I established the basis of relationship in the department: Everyone moves up. Everyone improves. Me too.

Later that week I asked, "By the way, Claudiu, what fellowship do you want?"

"Infectious diseases," he said. My own specialty.

Downstate was a school that had rarely kept any of its own students in the training program for residency. The people who knew us best liked us least. Later the same year, Downstate kept dozens of its own students in the training program for the first time ever. They felt comfortable enough to stay. The basis of the faculty's relationship with trainees was no longer managing the boss. It became achieving the goal of the group and making the best "product."

I chose to close this chapter with this story because is important for those trying to recruit and run training programs of any kind. Treating our newest graduates as the most qualified ever to come out of school is in society's best interest. It is in our best interest to recognize their superiority and to ask their assistance in developing medical advances and research. It is in our interest to honor the current graduate as the person who will find the cure for diseases we will all suffer someday.

PART 2

An Open Mind
Saves Lives

CHAPTER 3

An Evangelist of the Eye Spreads the Good Word

I N MY CLASSES, I like to discourage the idea that the teacher is all-knowing. If a student or resident can prove me wrong or tell me something I didn't know, I hand him or her a $5 or $10 bill. The same goes for patients. It's my way of making sure that I never stop learning. A physician should live as a perpetual student, open to learning even in the unlikeliest places.

Beryl Hamilton, a delightful 82-year-old woman who wore glasses for nearly 50 years, is an unlikely source of medical knowledge. I call her up, just wanting to talk to her on the phone for a few minutes. She offers to meet me at the hospital, immediately, now. She is a little irritated I didn't call the day before: "My doctor told me you would call. Why didn't you call yesterday? I want to tell you about this."

Ms. Hamilton suffered from cataracts, which are common in older people. The lens of the eye slowly becomes opaque. Less and less light passes through. Night vision goes first. The patient doesn't perceive extra-low light and finds it almost impossible to drive at night. In cataract surgery, the surgeon makes an incision around the base of the cornea, where it attaches to the sclera, the white part of the eye. The surgeon can put a small device through the incision and pop out the cataract, or he or she can put a small suction device inside the cornea, suck out the cloudy part, and insert a new lens. Removing the cloudy part still leaves the capsule of the lens intact. The process is like pulling out the filling in a jelly doughnut and putting a new filling inside.

Cataract surgery is the most common surgical procedure in the country. It wasn't so long ago that eye surgeons would make a 180-degree incision around the cornea, flap open the entire eye, and then just couch the affected lens.

"What do you mean by *couch the lens?*" I ask ophthalmology fellow Mohamed Hajee in an interview for this book.

"That means you just push it backward into the eye and leave it there," he replies.

"Are you kidding?" I ask. "Just shove it back?" The idea of couching a lens, like kicking your garbage under the sofa, strikes me as barbaric.

"Yes, you pushed it backward, and you were left without a lens, and you left the person wearing glasses that looked like the bottoms of coke bottles. These patients were also left with an increased risk of retinal detachment."

I guess this kind of cataract removal must have seemed like a major advance in its day—like the first typewriter, which weighed 800 pounds; or the first EKG machine, which two men had to carry on a hand truck; or early computers, whose eight megabytes took up an entire room. Small is the way of the future.

Mohamed Hajee says, "We put instruments into the eye that are amazingly small and less damaging to the tissue of the eye. Twenty-five-gauge surgery [surgery with a needle less than half the size of a needle used to draw blood] means you can shorten the operating time. The shorter a procedure is, the less the complications are. It used to take about forty-five minutes to do the surgery; now we do it with a two-millimeter incision in a procedure that takes four to seven minutes."

And there's no more couching, either, because now eye surgeons can insert a catheter into the lens and suck out the contents.

The replacement lenses are small, sharp, and highly functional. The cataract surgery not only restores the patient's sight but also improves it beyond the best eyesight he or she ever had. Virtually every form of human endeavor has improved over time, and the next generation is seen as the hope of something better.

Beryl Hamilton says that she is "high on mighty lenses" and that she wants to "convert" me.

"At first, I used to see a halo around bright objects," she says, describing her battle with cataracts. "Eventually, it progressed to the point where I could not see to write my own name. I would also have to spend a lot of money on glasses, because my eyes were getting worse over time. I was changing my glasses and spending close to five hundred dollars every two years to get the right prescription.

"I did not just have a new lens, young man, I had a ReSTOR lens. I used to have reading glasses and glasses for distance. I could not read a book. Now I see *everything*. I can read the finest print, and I can see far away. I am seeing wonderful! The ReSTOR lens makes it so I can read all the books I used to need special glasses to see before. My children say to me, 'Mommy, are you really reading that book, or are you just looking at it?' They can't believe I can see everything. They are so used to me wearing glasses. When I first got the ReSTOR lens, I went home and put on my old glasses. My vision was blurry when I put on my glasses! When I took off the glasses, my vision was clear."

"What's a ReSTOR lens?" I ask.

Oh, now I have done it! Ms. Hamilton becomes a prophet of the prescription. An orator of ophthalmology. An evangelist of the eye. "You mean you never heard of the ReSTOR lens?" She does not say it in a judgmental way at all. She is an evangelist in the true meaning of the word, from the Greek *eu,* which means "good," and *angelos,* which means "news." She says, "The ReSTOR lens works like a bifocal. You see both near and far."

ReSTOR is the brand name of just one of these bifocal-type lenses.

There are others that do pretty much the same thing, such as a Crystalens or a ReZoom lens.

Ms. Hamilton continued, "When I see people with glasses on, I say, 'Why are you putting those things on your face?' After I had it done, I was reading on the bus, and a woman saw me reading the fine print in a book. She was reading over my shoulder. She asked me how I was able to see the fine print. I told her about the ReSTOR lens, and she went straight to my doctor to get one, and she does not even live near here. She lives in Washington, D.C., and works at the National Institutes of Health. She works at NIH, and she did not know about it!"

I do not even have cataracts, and Beryl Hamilton makes me want to go out and get my own ReSTOR lenses put in!

"Now I read better than I did when I had glasses on," she says in summary.

Keep going, Ms. Hamilton. Rub it in. You know something more than I do. I owe you $5 for the fact.

CHAPTER 4

"Practicing" Interventional Radiology

A Nearly Missed Treatment for Fibroids

DURING THE PAST decade, researchers developed a device that uses radiofrequency energy to tighten the lower esophageal sphincter in patients suffering from gastroesophageal reflux disease. Instead of performing surgery, physicians could use a scope to essentially scar and tighten the lower esophagus. Known as the Stretta procedure, it was a fantastic advance.

Dr. Frank Gress, Professor of medicine in the division of gastroenterology, asks me, "Do you know what happened with the Stretta procedure?"

I am about to say, "It eliminated ninety percent of surgery. It's a miracle," but he doesn't wait for me to answer.

"It failed. It was abandoned. The company went out of business."

Whoa! What's up with that?

"It was a great advance," he continues. "Reflux symptoms were resolved without the need for medications or surgery, by using a scope. But the company was unsuccessful in getting physicians or patients to change their behavior. The data was promising, but the company just couldn't sell the product. They went out of business because of lack of use."

Time and again I have heard of physicians and patients who have missed an important opportunity for healing because they were afraid to try something unfamiliar and new. Meanwhile, equipment that would be the envy of any science-fiction writer's brain sits gathering dust.

DID YOU EVER wonder why we say physicians are "practicing" medicine? Strange word, isn't it? You would think that with four years of college, four years of medical school, and a minimum of three years of residency for a basic specialty and seven years for advanced training, they wouldn't have to practice, they would have it mastered! In interventional radiology, you see the reason for the term: the standard of care is to be always learning something new.

Interventional radiology has replaced a lot of surgery. Instead of sending you to the operating room for a biopsy, interventional radiologists simply use a needle and then send you home. Instead of giving you general anesthesia, which carries risks, they simply give you a local shot to numb the area and a benzodiazepine medication like Valium to make you sleepy before they begin their work. Instead of slicing you open, they thread a catheter up the femoral artery. Although modern surgery is amazingly safe, with an error rate similar to transcontinental jet flight, operations still carry risk. That risk is markedly decreased by doing procedures without the need for scalpels and ventilators.

Dr. Sal Sclafani is chairman of radiology and chief of interventional radiology at SUNY Downstate School of Medicine. I am in his office conducting an interview with him for this book. "Tell me, Sal, what new thing have you brought to health care in the last few years?"

Sal, in his sixties, still exudes a youthful exuberance you might find in a Silicon Valley start-up company exec. He is the epitome of the modern wired man. I half expect him to start throwing a basketball in the office in order to think and to ponder. He has traveled around the world taking pictures, and his office is decorated with photo travel books. With a cheerful smile and a warm demeanor, he talks about the latest radiologic imaging methods underneath a salt-and-pepper ponytail that makes me wonder if he will interrupt our discussion to have a fish taco and go surfing.

"Before I tell you about the kid we brought back from the dead after being stabbed in the ear and head with a carving knife, let me tell you about uterine artery embolization," he says in answer to my question. "This is the single procedure I do most often. This is where a radiologist gets to feel like a primary care practitioner."

Uterine artery embolization (UAE), Sal explains, is a cutting-edge treatment for uterine fibroids, the most common lesion of the uterus. As many as 50 percent of women have these tumors. Many women carry them for years without symptoms, but when fibroids do become symptomatic, they present with bleeding that can often be severe. Periods last as long as ten days, and the intense bleeding soaks through many pads a day.

Sometimes fibroids are so large that they press on the bladder, which can make a woman have to get up two or three times a night to urinate. Then, of course, many women get severe pain from the lesions as well. Hormonal therapy can be effective, but it can lead to mood changes and emotional irritability. The standard of care for many years has been a hysterectomy, the surgical removal of the entire uterus. Besides the risks of the surgery and the general anesthesia, downsides to a hysterectomy include a recovery time of several weeks and the loss of reproductive potential. A UAE spares women these downsides. It involves putting a catheter into the femoral artery and threading it up into the arteries supplying the uterus, then injecting a sclerosing agent that will clog, or embolize, the artery.

THE CONTROL ROOM of the interventional radiology suite where Dr. Sal Sclafani works his miracles is the sacristy of the temple of modern medicine. Everything is shiny, new, and lovingly used: high-tech machines from floor to ceiling on every side, lead aprons to protect the male staff lest leaking radiation damages their sperm counts. But the air is not antiseptic; it holds the scent of the desire to be on the absolute cutting edge of technology. Faculty members ages 32 to 72 all know that being current in interventional radiology means being willing to accept that today's state-of-the-art procedures may have to be discarded by next year. Sal has invited me here today to observe a UAE procedure.

"We rarely get referrals from gynecologists," Sal says. "Most of our patients hear about the procedure by word of mouth." Sal is being politic here, obliquely referring to the fact that gynecologists are surgeons in the business of doing gynecologic surgery; they are not in the business of embolizing the blood supply to the uterus with a needle. As chair of an enormous department of radiology that covers three hospitals in New York City, he knows how to make his point without offending his colleagues.

But, as his patient this morning, Alison R., says, "I saw two gynecologists for my bleeding, and neither of them told me about this procedure. They told me that surgery to remove my uterus was the only way to control my bleeding if medications did not work."

In the control room today are people who work daily with radiation in order to serve and protect patients. A technician, Ben, is standing next to me. He has on a lead apron as well as a lead necklace that protects his thyroid. "You should see the cool procedure the neuroradiologist does to stop aneurysms in the brain," he says. "That would be great for your book."

ALISON HAS HAD abnormal vaginal bleeding for the last two years. Every one of her periods saw enormous increases in bleeding. Prior to observing the procedure, I interview Alison and her partner of 12 years, David.

Alison, a schoolteacher, tells me that she once had to have someone come into her class to cover so that she could run to the bathroom and change her pads. If she stood up after sitting for a long time, blood would come gushing out, which was especially bothersome after driving to work. She had to take days off, often two or three at a time, sometimes every month. I can see how much this bothers her.

"The hardest thing about having fibroids and bleeding," she says, "is that I pride myself on being a strong woman. I do everything right. I exercise, I am a vegetarian, and I am strong. It is so embarrassing to have to feel weak because I had bleeding from my vagina that I could not control."

Her doctor offered no hope. "I told my gynecologist that surgery was not an option for me," she says. "I really could not take three weeks off work in the middle of the school year. My gynecologist never told me about this procedure."

Physicians are so focused on their own specialty that they are often ignorant of what is going on in other disciplines, but what Allison says next makes it obvious that hers was still living in the dark ages. "I told him I was looking into other methods. His response was flippant. He said, 'If you want to try acupuncture or whatever else, that's fine, but don't call me when you hemorrhage again!' I had bleeding so bad sometimes that I had to go the emergency department. I felt lucky because I wasn't having pain. But I was getting light-headed."

David says, "We tried hormonal therapy with progesterone, but her mood changed a lot. She became very irritable. She would make a big deal about something small. She would carry on longer than she normally would. Alison saw this and said, 'I can't believe I went on so long about something stupid.'"

"How else did you feel?" I ask Alison.

"I felt ashamed," she replies. "I pride myself on being a very healthy person. It was embarrassing having something wrong with me. I did not feel like me."

"How did you find out about this procedure?"

"Not from my doctor. One knew about it but told me it was not a good idea."

There it is again, that medieval fear of the strange and unfamiliar, alive and well in 21st-century medicine.

"We found out about it at a health fair," Alison says.

David explains that the bleeding has ranged from inconvenient to disabling. "Alison likes to go dancing, but she really gets nervous about it now because of the bleeding. It might soak through her clothes and she gets really embarrassed, but I don't care. I know it bothers her. We were at dinner and had to leave suddenly because the bleeding got so bad."

His love is so obvious. He simultaneously makes it clear that this is a disabling condition for her, but he will not show the slightest sense of being bothered by it himself. His acceptance and unconditional love are palpable. "She has had to wear those diapers, Depends, you know," he says. "But I don't mind. Alison has shown so much love for me for the ten years before, and has taken such good care of me, that it is just an inconvenience for me. Besides that, nothing could scare me away from the love I have for Alison."

SHOSHANA ELLENBERG, SHANA for short, is the coordinator of the uterine artery embolization program. She is a stylishly dressed, elegant woman taking care of a messy disease. She meets Alison before the procedure to go over the details. I inspect Shana's information sheets regarding Alison.

> Bleeding amount: Enormous
> Frequency: Often
> Pads used daily: Numerous
> Days of bleeding: Nine days a month

I ask what other procedures Shana coordinates.

"Just these," she says. "This is a full-time job all by itself."

"Are you Orthodox?" I ask.

"Very much!" the effervescent Shana says, smiling.

A huge understanding suddenly opens between us. In Orthodox

Judaism there is a strict prohibition on physical contact—any contact, even so much as a kiss, a hug, or holding hands—between a man and a woman during menstrual flow and for five days afterward.

Shana explains, "It might lead to sexual contact, so even so much as touching fingers is forbidden."

Shana and I joke around. "So getting rid of the fibroids means adding another week of sex!" I say, smiling. A new enormity hits me: an Orthodox woman with a fibroid might not be able to touch her husband for half the month.

"Yup," she replies, "a good time to go on vacation!"

Smiles all around, smiles and laughs. But she and I both know what this means. Having fibroids is more than an inconvenience or embarrassment; it leads to a terrible loss of intimacy. I gratefully move back to the details of the program before we can ponder how horrible it must be to lose all physical contact with the man you love for as much as half the month.

I stand behind lead-impregnated glass to see the patient and the monitor as the UAE procedure begins. I see the outline of the uterus and its intricate arboretum of blood vessels. Dr. Sal Sclafani carefully places the catheter in each of the supplying vessels and shoots a little contrast, or dye, in each of them to make sure of the target before he injects the agent that will embolize the artery.

I hear Sal talking to Alison. "I am not going to cut you," he says. "I will not use a knife. I am going to look at each of the vessels to see which are supplying the fibroids, and then I will clog them off. You will be uncomfortable for a few hours, but you will be able to go home tonight. About eighty-five percent of patients see an enormous improvement in their bleeding in general, but I see a better response even than that."

And no recovery time! I think.

When I talk to Dr. Sclafani about it afterward, he says that, no, patients still experience about six hours of discomfort or pain after the UAE procedure. I have to laugh. My own simple hernia repair the year before was only a 30-minute procedure, but it left me with difficulty walking for days. I needed a catheter in the site for days to directly inject anesthetic so that I would not be incapacitated. Even now I had discomfort when I exercised or stood for a long time.

What a wonderful world, where fibroid sufferers can choose six hours of recovery time over the weeks it takes to recuperate from a hysterectomy.

Eighteen minutes after it starts, the procedure is over. The artery is embolized. Alison, sleepy but cheerful, is taken to the recovery room. There is a huge sense of relaxation and freedom in her facial expression. Alison has only another hour or two to wait before David takes her home from a same-day procedure with a nearly 90 percent chance of getting better.

David reaches his hand through the side rails to touch her arm. "David makes me feel very comfortable. I am a very fortunate woman," Alison says. Her happiness is palpable despite the momentary discomfort.

CHAPTER 5

Resistance Is Futile

Safe Surgery for Spines

FAYVERLYN MILLER IS crying when she tells me about the pain she was in. "They sent me to a pain management specialist. They sent me for acupuncture. They sent me to a chiropractor. They sent me for rehabilitation. They sent me to a psychiatrist!"

For nearly a decade, "they" sent her for everything except an MRI and an evaluation for spinal surgery by Dr. Mike Gerling, a specialist in minimally invasive spinal procedures at SUNY Downstate. Once she did find her way to his office, Dr. Gerling discovered that one of Ms. Miller's vertebrae had slipped forward onto another, a condition called spondylolisthesis. It can be tremendously painful, because instead of the pressure going from bone to bone, the pressure smashes down on the nerve roots. It is like your hand being slammed in a car door.

Dr. Gerling promised relief, but, Ms. Miller says, "People tried to warn me off doing the back surgery. People said, 'What do you want to go messing with your back for?'"

"People have a legitimate fear," says Dr. Gerling.

The paraspinal muscles are huge, and traditionally the only way to fixate a bone was to make a huge cut and fillet off the muscle. The very

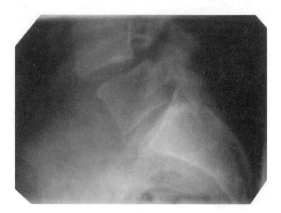

*Spondylolisthesis: the spine with the
vertebra on top slipped forward.*

act of moving and manipulating the muscles causes enormous trauma
to them, no matter how careful you are. They atrophy.

Stronger back muscles improve back pain. The stronger the muscles
of your back, the more they carry the load and the less dependent the
body is on the bones of the spine. Dr. Gerling says, "You don't care about
having the disc removed. You worry about me tearing the muscles apart,
you worry about nerve roots being damaged."

People say it's getting harder and harder to write good science fiction
at the rate that science and technology are advancing.

"There is a lot of new technology," Dr. Gerling acknowledges, "but
we have had a lot of learning to do to figure out what to do with it.
We have a lot of new tools and toys. Sometimes when you have a new
technology, you don't know how to use it for a while. The ultimate
outcome is not groundbreaking, but the way we achieve the outcome
has entirely changed. We do things smaller now. What is changed is
how we *get* to the spine."

Fear is a significant barrier to spinal surgery. The smaller the surgery, the smaller the fear.

"The biggest question," says Dr. Gerling, "is, How do we reach the
bone? Instead of going down the midline and stripping the muscle off

the bone, we can make a very small incision, less than two centimeters, to operate through. We can put in a little dilator and operate through a tube to take out the disc." He describes the instrument used in such operations as a thin little bayonet forceps. "I am doing the surgery looking at a TV screen," he adds. "You can pull a massive piece of disc out of the spinal canal that was crushing all the nerve roots, and you don't have to traumatize all the muscles around the spine," he explains. "The patients can literally get up the day after their procedure and touch their toes."

This technology has existed for years, but it "arrived" only recently. I ask Dr. Gerling why it has taken so long for us to accept operating through tubes instead of filleting open the paraspinal muscles.

He says, "Most spine surgeons don't do this type of surgery. There is an advantage to being operated on by someone who has graduated from training relatively recently ... If you are a successful spine surgeon for the last twenty years, you are not going to embrace that new technology. Your whole eye-hand coordination was never trained to operate through a tube or to look through an arthroscope at a TV monitor. It's completely different. You are not looking directly at the bone that is open and exposed. You are not putting a piece of metal directly on bone that you can touch and scrape. You would not take the time out of your practice for the many months or years it would take to retrain your eye-hand coordination. You are not going to embrace that new technology. You are used to pulling back the muscles five centimeters off the bone. That's why there is an advantage to being operated on by someone trained recently. Patients don't have as much blood loss, they don't have as much volume loss, and they are not lying there on massive amounts of opiates."

This is not just a change in procedure; it is also a change in thought. The patient's comfort and safety are now important considerations. Patients no longer need to be afraid. On the other hand, Dr. Gerling is the only physician performing this procedure in all of Brooklyn, one of the largest cities in the country. Most spine surgeons were trained in earlier eras. The fear that Fayverlyn Miller and other spine patients experience makes it urgent for more new physicians to enter the field.

Ms. Miller was seen by at least four doctors before she got an appropriate diagnosis.

"The pain was going on for eight or nine years," she says. "I am a single mother and I always worked. I was never out of a job. Now I couldn't work, I had no income, and this was devastating. I got cortisone injections, but it made no difference, and the pain was getting worse and worse over time. Acupuncture and two chiropractors also made no difference."

Ms. Miller waited desperately for a physician to come along who would listen with an open mind. "I was so angry. My life became smaller and smaller. I couldn't do anything." I ask, "What sort of impact did it have on your daily life?"

She replies, "I could not stand up to wash the dishes, I could not stand long enough to take a shower. When I was walking, I had to stop every three or four minutes to take a break."

In Brooklyn neighborhoods, people walk everywhere: to the store, the dry cleaner, a friend's house. When walking down the street, like a shipwreck survivor reaching for any floating piece of wood to save herself from drowning. Ms. Miller had to stop and sit on the front stoops of strangers. I ask her if it was the pain or shortness of breath that forced her to sit.

"Pain, pain, the pain, the pain!" she says emphatically. "The most frightening thing is that I thought I was going to end up in a wheelchair. I had three aunts with back pain that got so bad they eventually ended up in wheelchairs." She starts to cry. "I was beginning to have to walk with a cane. I was very depressed; I started to use antidepressant medications. The worst thing was that the doctors were not believing the amount of my pain, and all they would do is give me more and more Motrin. I kept saying, 'Something is wrong, something is truly wrong,' but they kept giving me Motrin and sending me back to the clinic. The biggest emotional impact was the doctor not believing my pain . . . Oh, I was so rude to them; at least I was ruder than I would normally be."

Here was a woman who could not stand to do her dishes or take a shower, yet she considered it rude to tell her doctors they were wrong.

Mike Gerling understands Ms. Miller's frustration. "One of the new dimensions in orthopedics is to start looking at the patient perspective of what we do," he says.

This might seem strange. If orthopedists have not been looking at procedures from the patient's perspective, then from exactly whose perspective have they been looking at it?

Dr. Gerling says, "Ten or fifteen years ago, it was rare to have validated measures of patient satisfaction. Now we can look at the profession from outside and figure out how to guide our therapy. A lot of patients were intimidated by their spine surgeon. They would tell the surgeon they were fine, but when they talked to other people they would say they were miserable. They would tell their doctor they were very satisfied with the procedure, but then they would need enormous amounts of narcotic medications to control their pain."

Fayverlyn Miller says, "When I met Dr. Gerling, now I figured I had one doctor who was working with me. They would not do the MRI before. They kept using all this medical terminology and treating me like I was stupid. I used to pray, 'Please send somebody who would understand what was going on.'"

To anyone with unexplained pain, she says not to stop questioning doctors: "You keep on them. You let them know the pain you are in . . . There will be one that will make a difference. Do not give up! If I had listened to them, I would be in a wheelchair right now."

DURING OUR INTERVIEW, Dr. Gerling gave me a thorough explanation of the new techniques for spinal surgery.

"Before," he says, "we would take bone grafts from the pelvis and put it into the patient's neck in order to get the bone grow together. People would wake up from their surgery, point to their pelvis, and say, 'It hurts there,' but feel okay at the spine. With our current technology, we don't have to do that. Now we have bone-bank bone."

Bone can be stored in a bone bank after being grown in a laboratory. The process begins with sucking out a sample of the patient's marrow, placing that sample in a centrifuge that isolates the stem cells for bone, and growing those cells in a culture. The doctor then collects the growing cells and slaps them onto the weak areas in the patient's bone. Bone-bank bone fills in gaps and preserves proper articulation in joints.

As Dr. Gerling puts it, "We have chemical substances and plates that are put in place internally so that patients don't need an external collar. The spine is fixated internally. We have chemical substances to fuse the bone. We have an engineered biological chemical substance, bone morphogenic protein, that is used to form bone. The future is very, very promising.

"We can use cadaver bone—an allograft—instead of harvesting it from another part of the person's body. I don't know if that seems exciting to other people, but it is exciting to your patients because it is so much less painful. It allows us to do shorter surgery. We can get in there and out much faster."

Dr. Gerling shows me contrasting pictures of patients operated on the old way and the new way. A fusion done his way leaves a small incision. A woman who before the operation could barely walk gets up and walks out of the hospital the following day with a cane, as opposed to five days later with a walker.

He shows me a video he has done of a patient the day after her spinal surgery. "Look at how obese this person is," he says. "Can you imagine a standard spine surgeon having to pull off nine centimeters of muscle to open the area? The ultimate end point is the same, but how we do it is so much better. I don't have to directly look at the open area. I do it through fiber-optic technology. I did not have to make another incision on the other side of this woman to operate on the other side. I put a little fiber-optic tube across the other side. I did not have to cut the skin on the other side. I did not have pull off all the muscles on the other side. The muscle does not get cut or torn."

Instead of laboring to stand, the woman in the video is walking on her own.

AFTER HER SURGERY with Dr. Gerling, Fayverlyn Miller says, "I have a whole new life now . . . Half the pain went away overnight, and it is still getting better and better."

I asked her what she was able to do afterward.

"They were amazed that I could walk the day after my surgery," she replies. "I can walk now. It's only three months since the surgery. I am extremely relieved. I now get to do things with my grandson. I can take him for walks. Before, I had to walk leaning to one side. Now everyone saw I was walking straight." She starts to cry a little with relief that she has not ended up in a wheelchair. "I was only in the hospital for three days, but I was up and walking the next day after the surgery. Now I don't have to sit on someone's stoop just to make it down the street." She wraps up by saying, "I know that me feeling better made Dr. Gerling feel better. He used to say to me, 'Don't cry, we will do what we can for you.'"

YOUNG DOCTORS TODAY seem to be more professional and less cynical than doctors of my generation. Don't expect anyone else to express this. Older docs are too busy talking about their previous superiority. When I was an intern, it was socially acceptable and even fully expected to burn out on actual patient care. It probably had to do with the toughness of our training, working 36-hour shifts and never calling in sick. Twice as a trainee I stuck myself with needles while attending to HIV-positive patients after I had been up for 24 hours. In those moments, I despised the patients I was working with. I confessed to one of my teachers,

"I just feel beaten. Every time my beeper goes off, I feel like I am being slapped."

He said, "It's okay; you will get your compassion back when you finish training."

I have never heard current trainees have to discuss compassion and empathy with faculty; it's just part of their culture. Program Directors, however, still regularly lament the "weakening" of training they perceive from limiting duty hours to a hamane and sane level.

GRACE MILLINER IS a 52-year-old woman who, like Fayverlyn Miller, had to rest on strangers' stoops just to walk down the block. Ms. Milliner did not get surgery for some time after her spondylolisthesis diagnosis because the hospital would not take her insurance.

"I was miserable, I was in such pain," she says. "I would have to go to the emergency department, and they would give me a shot, which would last for a few days, but then it would go right back. I couldn't sleep because I couldn't lie down right. I would sleep for two hours and then wake up in pain. I couldn't bend over, and I could not stand up to do my dishes. I felt like a cripple. I couldn't make my bed, I couldn't carry my laundry. I couldn't entertain people in my house."

Managed care strikes again, and it makes me angry. Nevertheless, Ms. Milliner says that she never gave up hope. I ask her what happened after the surgery.

"I can dance!" she exclaims. "I can wind my waist." Then she giggles like a teenager. "I am one hundred percent better. I can touch my toes. I got a whole new life."

I say, "You must be really happy."

"I am on cloud nine!"

MS. JEANNETTE ESCOBAR is a 44-year-old woman who describes excruciating back pain: "It progressed to the point that I couldn't even move. It was the lowest of the low. I couldn't even do anything. I went for acupuncture, I tried nerve stimulation electrically, and I got cortisone shots. The shots would only last one or two days. I went to see my doctor, and he wanted to do an MRI, but it was a month before the test was approved. I couldn't sleep throughout the night.

"I got sent to a pain management doctor, but it didn't help. It was so frustrating. I could not stand for a long period of time, I couldn't shop even for small things because I couldn't walk up and down the aisle. Then I would sit, but I couldn't do that for a long period of time either. I would have to lean against the wall to straighten my back. I couldn't walk. I had to cut down my showers to less than ten minutes because of the pain. I worked in a day care center, and I could not do my job. I did not visit anybody. I thought I was disabled. I was only forty-four years old. I thought, 'I am too young for this to happen.' I thought I had no right to be like this, and I was very mad about it."

After a few months, the pain management doctor told Ms. Escobar that he could do nothing more for her and suggested that she see a surgeon. She then contacted Dr. Mike Gerling.

"When I got the procedure on Monday, I went home on Tuesday night," she says. "As soon as I got into the recovery room, I could start to move my legs. Now all I have left is a little pain when I wake up in the morning, but that is it."

She and I talk about the fear people have of back surgery.

"I put my trust in my doctor," she says. With the new, smaller, less invasive procedure, she was not afraid of muscle trauma and atrophy, nor was she worried about nerve roots being damaged.

Ms. Escobar exclaims, "Thank you for giving me my life back!"

CHAPTER 6

An Open Mind Saves Lives

New Techniques in Gastroenterology

REFLUX IS STOMACH acid that comes up into the esophagus, causing a lot of pain, coughing, hoarseness, and even cancer. It's one of the most common illnesses that gastroenterologists see. Reflux disease makes the esophagus more like a stomach. After a few years, acid exposure changes the histology, or cell type, of the esophagus, a condition called Barrett's esophagus, which can transform into cancer at a rate of about 0.5 percent a year. Dr. Frank Gress, who you met in chapter 4, tells me, "We used to have to take all those patients to the operating room to remove the end of the esophagus, which would pull up the stomach and eliminate half the stomach."

Surgery was the only option until 2005, when Frank started using radiofrequency ablation (RFA) to remove early stage esophageal cancer. RFA allows us to scrape off the precancerous cells in your esophagus without the slightest cut. "With surgery," he says, "you would have to stay in the hospital for five days, then go home for another month's recovery. Then the long-term recovery is adjusting to not having a stomach anymore. With surgery, you can't eat like you used to. You get dumping syndrome. Your whole way of life changes." Dumping syndrome is the rapid release of food into the intestines from having a stomach that is too small. It causes light-headedness and shaking. It is really uncomfortable and has no cure. You manage it by never eating a big meal. Never. For the rest of your life.

Radiofrequency ablation, performed through an endoscope, eliminates the need for cutting out the bottom third of your esophagus, yanking your stomach up into your chest, and then reattaching it to your esophagus. "How long is the recovery time?" I ask, thinking about how so much of 21st-century medicine has been about achieving objectives with less damage. "You have the procedure and go home that day. In a few days you are back to normal," says Frank.

"How much longer does it take than a regular endoscopy?"

"About fifteen minutes."

"Wow," I say, "a whole fifteen or twenty minutes extra." No reaction on Frank's face. I'm pleading, "Would you look happy for a second, please?" Frank Gress is not a dour person. He normally exudes enormous personal warmth. "Come on, Frank, give me the 'happy look'!" He smiles and laughs. Maybe high-level problem solvers like him have such high expectations that their satisfaction can't last. Maybe these advancements are all in a day's work to them. Maybe Dr. Gress just needs reminding that prior to his arrival, Downstate — the only medical school in Brooklyn — could not offer *any* of these advanced procedures. He laughs some more. I say into my tape recorder: "Frank is looking happy now."

But only for a moment. "We haven't been doing a lot of them here yet. We need to do a lot of education in the community. Doctors are trained to think that if you have high-grade dysplasia, which turns into cancer, then you should go see a surgeon. The surgeon will happily take out your esophagus. This culture has to change." Now Frank is back to looking weary. After an English physician named James Lind prescribed limes and other citrus fruits to prevent scurvy in the mid-18th century, it took the British navy 40 years to stock its ships with them. In 1867, British surgeon Joseph Lister proved that antiseptic, sterile surgery cut the death rate by 80 percent. Yet it took him most of the next 20 years to convince surgeons to wash their hands and put on sterile gloves. Physicians take a long time to change, particularly in procedure-based specialties. This is why patient advocacy is so important. Physicians tend not to see patient demands as a good thing. Some still think, *Who are they to question my judgment?* A disappointing number of physicians choose to order procedures based on what they know and are comfortable with, rather than learn what's new.

Surgical procedures to control reflux by tightening up the lower esophagus have been in use for 50 years. Proton pump inhibitors have been used for nearly 20 years to control acid production. A few years ago, a device was developed to use radiofrequency energy to tighten the lower esophageal sphincter. Instead of performing surgery, physicians could use a scope to essentially scar and tighten the lower esophagus. Known as the Stretta procedure, it was a fantastic advance. Frank asks me, "Do you know what happened with the Stretta procedure?" I am about to say, "It eliminated ninety percent of surgery; it's a miracle," but he doesn't wait for me to answer. "It failed. It was abandoned. The company went out of business." Whoa! What's up with that?

"It was a *great* advance," says our professor of gastroenterology. "Reflux symptoms resolved without the need for medications or surgery, by using a scope.". But guess what. "The company was unsuccessful in getting physicians or patients to change their behavior. The data was promising, but the company just couldn't sell the product. They went out of business because of lack of use."

Instead of undergoing open surgery or taking daily medications for the rest of your life, you could have had a simple procedure, "like a suntan that tightens up and thickens the lower esophagus," according to Frank. Abandoned due to lack of use. Turns out patients would rather take medications, and doctors just want to do what they know.

THE 18-YEAR-OLD WOMAN in the bed at Kings County Hospital has terrible diarrhea with blood and abdominal pain. She might have an infection inside her abdomen as well. She also has a hole between her intestines and her vagina. Stool is coming out of her vagina because of the abnormal hole, called a fistula. Her illness, Crohn's disease, forms fistulae with any part of the body that a loop of bowel might be touching. Often this is between two loops of bowel. Sometimes it is between the bowel and the bladder, and stool comes out in the urine. Sometimes it is between a loop of bowel and the anterior abdominal wall, so that the sufferer passes liquid stool through multiple places in the skin.

I imagine my own personal life, with all its fears and anxieties, and then I imagine being a young woman trying to explain to her boyfriend something like a rectocutaneous fistula or stool coming from her vagina. Imagine having bags attached to your abdomen to deposit liquid, horribly malodorous stool. Sometimes the bags leak and make the room smell foul. Suddenly whatever fears I have in a relationship are small in comparison.

Crohn's disease is a very severe form of inflammatory bowel disease. Inflammatory cells known as granulomas can form anywhere in the inner walls of the gastrointestinal tract, from the mouth to the anus. The granulomas of Crohn's disease can create a connection with whatever they touch and pierce the wall of the guts. Crohn's disease is incurable.

Crohn's disease and its related disorder, ulcerative colitis, used to make the person waste away until he or she died—essentially of malnutrition. Thirty years ago there wasn't much at all to be done. Long after my mother got divorced, she had a serious boyfriend named Frank. I still remember sitting in the backseat of the car at 12 or 13 and watching them hold hands in an ocean of peaceful communion. Unlike my father, Frank respected my mother, opened the car door for her, lit her cigarettes, never ate without her eating first, helped her into her coat, and was infinitely reverential. One day Frank got sick. I ended up accompanying my mother to the hospital. Her big dark glasses were on, the kind that hide crying and dark circles. Frank had inflammatory bowel disease, or colitis. Steroids didn't control his dozens of bowel movements a day. Even with total parenteral nutrition through a central line in his jugular vein, he weighed 90 pounds. Total parenteral nutrition can't replace the calories and muscle mass a patient loses with uncontrolled inflammatory bowel disease. "He brought me back to life after leaving your father. I had never been treated well before," says my mother. "By the time they tried to remove his colon for the colostomy to stop the colitis, he was too debilitated, and he died." I did not find out until after he died that my mother was going to marry him.

If this story had taken place only 20 years later, it might have had a happy ending instead of a tragic one. Today we have oral medications such as mesalamine derivatives that are quite useful in controlling the disease. When I met the very unfortunate 18-year-old woman with Crohn's disease, mesalamine was helping her. It was my first day at Kings County Hospital, and I was learning about the new patients.

"What are we doing for this lady?" I asked the medical team.

"Intravenous antibiotics, mesalamine, and steroids," one said.

"What about infliximab?" I asked.

"No one said to do that."

This infuriating attitude is one of the biggest problems in medicine. If the subspecialist, who is supposed to know *more* than you, does not tell you to do something, he or she must be right.

"I don't care what they say, let's try," I said. The days of blindly following authority in medicine have got to end. Crohn's disease is as rare as reflux disease is common, but both demand that physicians keep an open mind.

Infliximab is a medication used to close fistulae. It is a genetically engineered antibody made in huge amounts to destroy a specific antigen: tumor necrosis factor. We started infliximab. In 48 hours, the patient's diarrhea and pain stopped. Another day or two later, and the fistula into her vagina closed! It is hard to imagine a more life-changing advance than infliximab in fistulizing Crohn's. Whenever I bring this up to gastroenterologists, they torture me by saying, "It doesn't work in everybody." So what? Let's focus on the fact that it works in two-thirds of people, and work on finding something else for the others.

DR. SCOTT TENNER is president of the New York State Society for Gastrointestinal Endoscopy and the governor of the American College of Gastroenterology. He publishes 50 times a year while running a huge private practice. Dr. Tenner travels the world — from Bombay to Boston, from Delhi to Detroit — to educate gastroenterologists in new procedures and new ways of thinking. Scott is also a skilled and dedicated lobbyist, visiting Washington to advocate for universal health coverage for colon cancer screening so that everyone has the opportunity to have a colonoscopy, thereby preventing 95 percent of deaths from this cancer.

One hundred fifty thousand Americans are diagnosed with colon cancer each year. Fifty thousand of them will die without the right detection. At the same time, there has been an explosion of treatments and diagnoses in gastroenterology. More methods of scoping the intestine have been developed in the last ten years than in the last half century of research and experimentation combined. Thirty years have passed since the development of the flexible fiber-optic endoscope. We have highly trained endoscopists who are able to detect and prevent nearly all of these deaths: 45,000 of America's 50,000 colon cancer deaths a year are preventable by colonoscopy. But we have yet to see a referendum on coverage for universal screening.

Scott is seeking funding to educate the public about the critical need to have a colonoscopy. Your risk of colon cancer is 6 to 8 percent in your lifetime. Dr. Tenner wants a massive advertising campaign to alert everyone to this and the means to do something about it: universal access to colonoscopy. He is "perfecting the world," removing obstacles to the right thing to do. He is one of the great men of our time.

Fear is the biggest barrier to the colonoscopy test. I am in the procedure room at Scott's private practice in Brooklyn when he tells me, "Propofol [a short-acting anesthetic] is a *miracle* of medicine"—not knowing what the title of this book will be. "The most important thing is the ability to put someone to sleep so I can do my procedure." The right anesthesia eliminates an enormous amount of the fear. "The patient has to wake up quickly. If the procedure and anesthesia are slow, far fewer people can be screened both for logistical reasons and for the elimination of the fear barrier. Waking up quickly, feeling well with your colonic polyp—an embryonic cancer—removed, is key to effective screening. The patient will wake up and say, 'Wow! That was a great sleep!' It is not like the old anesthesia where people were groggy or uncomfortable. This anesthesia does not go too far to the point where the patient needs to be intubated. People are comfortable."

Although the outcome might be the same as it was 20 or 30 years ago, the experience of a colonoscopy has changed entirely. This is not just a change in procedure, however; it is also a change in thought. The patient's comfort and safety are now important considerations. Scott Tenner's passion is for the person, not the lab results. Detecting disease—and curing it—is only part of the experience now, for both doctor and patient.

Scott is bothered by my recitation of the all the great stuff I have learned about the practice of gastroenterology so far, such as the celiac block, radiofrequency ablation of early esophageal dysplasia, and the endoscopic mucosal resection (EMR) of gastrointestinal tumors. "What more remarkable miracle do you want than being able to prevent ninety-five percent of colon cancer?" he asks me.

"You think you can prevent ninety-five percent of colon cancer?"

He practically screams, "I don't *think* we can prevent ninety-five percent of colon cancer, I *know* we can do it!"

Scott's emotions are shocking. He is usually a very smooth and unflappable Harvard-trained gastroenterologist. He shouts, "What more do you want as a miracle of modern medicine?! Think of all the suffering we can prevent, think of the surgery we can prevent, think of all the chemotherapy that patients won't have to use! You, in your lifetime, may not get EMR, you may not get a celiac block, but you have a six to eight percent chance of colon cancer, which can be prevented. Isn't that enough for you?! We start scoping at 7:00 A.M. and finish at 7:00 P.M. at night, but the truth is, we should be going to midnight every night."

Colonoscopy is not a new procedure. But the concept of near disease elimination for cancer is new. Although Scott Tenner is a leading national expert on all things in the gastrointestinal tract, his major global contribution is when he is lobbying to expand the public's access to colonoscopy. This is when his passion flares. This is when he is my hero.

Physicians are conservative by nature. This may be partly why physicians, at least in the past, have been some of the most vocal opponents of universal health care coverage. The idea of change makes us nervous. For a doctor, universal coverage calls to mind the specter of socialized medicine, which he or she takes to mean shortchanging the doctor and interfering in his or her control of medicine. Nothing scares the doctor more than the possibility of eliminating choices for both the patient and the physician and adding another layer of approval before doing what is medically necessary.

Now, however, physicians' groups such as the American Medical Association and the American College of Physicians have strongly and conclusively come out in support of reforming health care. They support the kind of lobbying it will take to make it happen, because universal coverage is an idea whose time has come. The *New England Journal of Medicine* has published editorial after editorial on the need for the leap to this form of social justice. Physicians and their leaders must not contribute to the inertia of the status quo. Maybe people like Scott Tenner, who for years has fought to make a safe, comfortable, rapid colonoscopy readily accessible to every American, will finally get their way. Perhaps Scott Tenner will soon be able to stop lobbying and claim a victory over colon cancer.

CHAPTER 7

What You Won't See on the Front Page

Reversing Strokes

ONE DAY I ask a laboratory technician what he thinks medicine's most exciting procedures are.

"Have you met Dr. Mangla?" the technician replies.

"Who?"

"Dr. Mangla. He is an interventional neuroradiologist."

"A what?"

"Interventional neuroradiologist. He removes clots from the brain with a catheter."

"What do you mean, 'removes clots from the brain with a catheter'? I've never heard of that."

Fifteen minutes later, I am shaking hands with Dr. Sundeep Mangla, a jaunty, articulate, balding man with the faint trail of a goatee and mustache that is unusual in academic medicine and research. Physicians, particularly outside private practice, don't generally possess a sense of personal style. In fact, personal style can be considered a liability in the sober, fact-based world of academic medicine, as if you can't be charming and accurate at the same time. Mangla, however, is both.

His "oh-great-that's-cool" persona doesn't seem worried about who I am as I thrust a voice recorder in his face and ask him to tell me the latest and coolest stuff about interventional neuroradiology, a subspecialty I first learned of a quarter of an hour ago.

As an advocate of being involved, I have to wonder why I have never heard of the procedures Sundeep Mangla carries out in my own institution. They are so amazing that I can't palm off my ignorance on his hiding in a corner of the hospital. Besides, I know from his first sentence that this is a man who is desperate for his work to be known. His desire to be known is not the egotistical kind that I get sometimes when someone higher up fails to acknowledge my accomplishments; rather, it is of the kind that says, "I have such good to do for you, if you will only let me tell you about it."

AN ISCHEMIC STROKE is caused by the obstruction of blood flow into parts of the brain. The obstruction results in rapid death of the tissue, because the brain has virtually no storage of oxygen or glucose. Even a few minutes of restricted blood flow can lead to cellular damage. After a few hours, the cells die and the damage is permanent. Sometimes this obstruction happens slowly as a clot forms in an artery in the brain. More often it happens quickly as a piece of clot flies off the heart to lodge in the brain. A clot in the brain that travels from somewhere else is called an embolus. One of the most common causes of emboli is an electrical rhythm disturbance in the heart known as atrial fibrillation. The blood doesn't flow rhythmically, and the stasis leads to the formation of a clot in the heart. The most common cause of atrial fibrillation is high blood pressure. High blood pressure is the most common disease in the United States, with about 60 million members in the club.

If you have high blood pressure that leads to atrial fibrillation that leads to a clot that leads to a stroke, you are likely to suffer severely impaired strength, speech, and sight. The weakness is almost always on one side of the body. If the stroke originated on the same side as the brain's speech center, you'd have difficulty talking. Ischemic stroke can also result in an instant coma or death.

When I was in training in the 1980s, neurologists were called to establish a diagnosis, and that was it; the benefits of neurology were therefore summarized as "diagnose and adios." This was particularly true in the management of stroke. I was not sure why we even called neurology, since, with rare exception, a diagnosis of stroke was obvious. A patient would come in with the sudden onset of weakness, numbness, difficulty speaking, or worse. We would get a CT scan of the brain, put the patient on an aspirin to inhibit blood clots, and call rehabilitation the next day to see what could be done to put Humpty Dumpty back together again. The answer was pretty uniform: nothing. The aspirin could only decrease the risk of another stroke; it couldn't do anything for the stroke at hand.

If the patient had atrial fibrillation, he or she was prescribed an anti-coagulant, or blood thinner, called warfarin (sold under the brand name Coumadin). For patients with atrial fibrillation, warfarin decreases the risk of stroke from about 5 to 6 percent a year to 2 to 3 percent a year. Like aspirin, warfarin does nothing for the current stroke; it only helps prevent the next one. As a side effect, warfarin also causes significant bleeding in about 1 percent of patients a year. The term *significant bleeding* refers to bleeding into your brain or bleeding bad enough to require a transfusion. Losing a cup of blood from your intestines does not count as significant (although, if you ask me, a cup of blood from my rectum is significant to me). One percent a year may not seem like a big number, but if it happens to you, it just won't matter to you that 99 percent of everyone else taking warfarin didn't have significant bleeding. It is 100 percent, because you are the only one of you that you have. Also, chances are 1 percent *a year*, so if you are 60 and need to be on warfarin for the rest of your life, each new year brings a new 1 percent chance of significant bleeding.

Another type of embolic stroke comes from a narrowed, or stenosed, carotid artery. Treatment for this type of stroke consists of filleting the carotid artery open from the top of the collarbone to the ear and stripping off the artery's inner layer. It is sort of like liposuction for the major artery going to the head. The mortality benefit of this treatment, called endarterectomy, is detectable only under very specific conditions. The narrowing must be more than 70 percent, and the patient has to live for at least five years for the benefit to become apparent. Just a little extra detail is that the vascular surgeon must have lots of experience doing this procedure; in anything except the best hands, the complication rate eliminates all evidence of mortality benefit. And, last but not least, endarterectomy, even in the hands of the best surgeon in the world, does nothing for the current stroke; it only prevents the next one.

So, in sum, for decades we have been able to offer three standard treatments to prevent stroke from blocked vessels: aspirin, warfarin, and endarterectomy. More recently, we added two medicines—dipyridamole and clopidogrel—that prevent emboli by inhibiting platelets (the blood cells that initiate clotting). These were all great breakthroughs in stroke prevention, but a treatment for an actual stroke remained elusive.

Thrombolytics—from *thrombus* (clot) and *lytic* (dissolve, break up, or destroy)—are medications that dissolve clots. Doctors had been using them to treat myocardial infarction, or heart attacks, since the 1970s. In the 1990s, studies of thrombolytics also showed that they reversed weakness, visual loss, and abnormal speech in stroke victims. People who get thrombolytics soon after the onset of a stroke have their clots dissolved, resulting in improved neurologic deficits and decreased mortality. But, because brain tissue is delicate, the medications must be given right away. The brain, as I said earlier, does not store oxygen or glucose, so it is sensitive to the restriction of blood flow. In order to see a benefit, the victim needs to get the thrombolytics within three hours of the onset of symptoms. But less than 5 percent of stroke victims receive medical attention within three hours, because a stroke does not cause pain. People come to the hospital with weakness or numbness, and the onset of numbness is harder to pinpoint than the onset of pain.

Just when I've had about enough of saying "but," in comes Dr. Mangla like a hero from the 1966 science-fiction classic *Fantastic Voyage*. In the movie, a team of miniaturized doctors is injected into the bloodstream of a scientist who has an inoperable blood clot in his brain. The movie had a big effect on me as a kid. Now here is Dr. Mangla taking me on a fantastic voyage into the human brain with 21st-century instruments. He can travel down every branch and twist of the cerebral vasculature with noninvasive imaging that shows the precise dimension of every little nuance of the circulation. He can rotate the images 360 degrees and expand or diminish them to any degree. He virtually puts us in a blood vessel, and we travel down it like a car in an East River tunnel. With his fantastic technology, Dr. Mangla is able to help stroke patients who arrive outside the three-hour window for thrombolytics.

"For patients who come late," he says, "we can direct administration of tPA [tissue plasminogen activator, a thrombolytic] into the brain. The first thing we can do is to angioplasty the cerebral vessel—"

I interrupt. "You are doing *angioplasty* of the cerebral vessels?"

"Yeah, of course."

"Don't say 'Yeah, of course.' You make it sound like everyone knows!"

A more effective alternative to thrombolytics, which melt the clot, angioplasty is a mechanical technique in which the surgeon yanks the clot out of the vessel. It is a standard procedure for unblocking coronary arteries, but I had no idea we could do angioplasty of cerebral arteries.

Before I can get my dropped jaw shut, Dr. Mangla adds, "We also do vertebral arteries. There is a middle cerebral artery angioplasty that I did of a forty-year-old woman who is a United Nations peacekeeper with expressive aphasia [inability to speak] and right arm weakness that was progressively getting worse."

"Did it help?"

"Yeah! It stopped. Five years later, and it is still resolved. There was also a man who had angioplasty of his vertebral arteries that we did angioplasty on. He would get dysarthria [difficulty talking] that was also associated with quadriparesis [weakness of all four limbs]. Every time he stood up, he would faint. He could not get up to leave the hospital. We did an angioplasty and a stent of his vertebral artery. All his symptoms resolved."

For the first time, finally, I am hearing about approaches to actual, not projected, strokes. I'm thrilled! "Are you finding the intra-arterial tPA useful?" I ask.

"It depends on the size of the clot. I am using less tPA over time because we have mechanical removal devices. It is like snow in your driveway. If you have a few inches of snow, the tPA is like rock salt to dissolve the clot. It is slower. If you have a larger clot, it is like a foot of snow or ice in the driveway. You are not going to melt the snow with tPA. You need a snow blower or shovel. The MERCI catheter"—MERCI stands for Mechanical Embolus Removal of Cerebral Ischemia—"pulls out big clots. Thrombolytics soften it up and macerate the clot so you can pull it out with the catheter. The tPA is too slow, and the longer you take to revascularize, the more brain there is that is dying."

The MERCI catheter, Dr. Mangla explains, has a little corkscrew at the end that snares the clot and pulls it out. I have never before heard of it. Neither has any of the dozens of physicians I talk to in the wake of my interview with Dr. Mangla.

He continues with another example. "We had an eighty-seven-year-old lady who came into the emergency department losing consciousness with paralysis of all four limbs. We used the MERCI catheter to remove the clot from the basilar artery [a main artery going up the spinal cord from the neck into the base of the brain], and she woke up and all her paralysis resolved within the week, and she became normal and walked out of the hospital."

In the past, we would have given this lady an aspirin and seen her either die or go on to live a depressed life completely dependent on someone to feed, clothe, and bathe her. How could I not have known about this catheter?!

"Then, of course," Dr. Mangla says, "there is the Penumbra catheter. The catheter has a little bead at the tip and is attached to a little vacuum cleaner. With a rocking motion, you can break up the clot and suck it out. The bead at the end and the rocking motion macerate the clot."

Penumbra, in astronomy, refers to the shadow cast around a celestial object. I imagine the stroke as a shadow cast around the celestial object that is your brain. Within the last five to ten years, we have gone at warp speed from several therapies that only prevent the next clot from forming to four separate modalities for reversing current strokes: intra-arterial tPA, angioplasty of the middle cerebral artery and vertebral artery, the MERCI catheter, and the Penumbra catheter. It's astounding. They are all being done at my own workplace, and I had no idea.

Strokes affect 700,000 people a year. Along with heart attack and cancer, stroke is one of the top three causes of death in the United States. So why aren't Dr. Mangla and his peers on the front page? I'm not the only one who ought to have known about their advances; patients and doctors alike should all know. How would you know to take your mother to a particular hospital to have a procedure done that you do not even know exists? I ask my students the following question: "What is worse: the fact that there is nothing you can offer a patient, or that there is something you can offer but you don't know it exists?"

Throughout our conversation, Dr. Mangla keeps saying he has not done many of these procedures, but I sweep that away. Of course he has not done many. How could he do many, when no one knows they are available? I am the person who is the lead educator for the largest department in the hospital. How are people supposed to refer patients to him for procedures like acute stroke reversal with a MERCI catheter when I have not heard about them? I hope that whatever invisible scorekeeper there is in the universe does not consign me to the nether regions of hell for being ignorant.

The following day, I go to morning report in the Department of Medicine. With 40 students and residents in the room, I present the cases: person with stroke after three hours, middle cerebral artery stenosis and clot, vertebral artery stenosis with dysarthria and fainting. I ask the crowd what they would do to solve this. No one, not even the residents who had been there for all of medical school prior to residency, knows that we do intra-arterial tPA, cerebral artery angioplasty, or vertebral artery angioplasty. I'm spreading the word about what Sundeep Mangla can do, and this is only for starters. Wait until they hear what he can do for hemorrhagic strokes.

A hemorrhagic stroke, the other main type of stroke besides the ischemic stroke, is caused by an aneurysm, which is the weakened wall of a blood vessel. An aneurysm is like a spot that bulges out on a bicycle inner tube. Sometimes it is a little bulge off to the side; this is called a saccular aneurysm, since it forms a sac. Sometimes the entire length of the vessel is weak. Either way, you would not feel it if you had an aneurysm right now. At least not until it ruptures and you bleed into your brain.

The standard treatment for a ruptured aneurysm has been a procedure called arterial clipping. I learned about it from a neurosurgeon who thought performing a craniotomy and putting a clip on the artery were as easy as pie. He said, "All you have to do is cut through the skull, lift up the brain, and, *boom,* there it is! The circle of Willis! You put the little clip on, flop the brain down, and put the skull back in place."

"Gee," I said to him, "I guess it's like sitting on the couch and losing your keys in the cushions. Just lift up the cushion, pick up the keys, and flop the cushion back in place."

The guy looked like he had just spent years in therapy with his mother and finally felt understood for the first time in his life. I was happy he felt so relieved. My comment was intended to be sarcasm, but he said, "That's it! Great! You got it!"

"Yeah, I got it," I said. "It's easy, except for one thing."

"What's that?"

"It's my brain, man!" I said, and walked away.

In our interview for this book, Sundeep Mangla tells me, "We can place a platinum wire into the aneurysm from the inside and plug up the aneurysm without having to cut open the skull or cut the brain. This greatly reduces the risk of an open surgical procedure. All the patient sees is a one-millimeter incision in the groin."

Using the platinum wire to plug up the aneurysm, a process called coiling, results not only in less bleeding than surgery but also in a much smaller chance of seizures. The destination is the same: prevent a blood vessel from bursting in your brain. But how do you travel in style? You can have someone chop pieces of your skull out. Or you can slip a catheter up the femoral artery in the groin and into the brain, where a little platinum-wire plug coils up in the aneurysm; then you pull out the catheter, leaving the coil in place. It is like stuffing up a rat hole with steel wool.

"People can immediately return to their productive lives with no noticeable change in them from the procedure," notes Dr. Mangla. "Subarachnoid hemorrhage [bleeding in the layer of blood vessels between the brain and its outer covering] is a clear area in which we use a catheter to block off the site of the ruptured aneurysm, save their lives and eventually get them back to a productive life."

"Save their lives" isn't a phrase you hear much in medicine. It has a very clear, pointed tone, and few physicians will use it. However, Dr. Mangla can use it with certainty in this case. He tells me, "We have a clear trial that shows that coiling the platinum wire in the aneurysm to block it off results in a 23 to 30 percent decrease in rebleeding compared with surgical clipping. This is an absolute risk reduction of 7.3 percent. That means you only have to do fifteen procedures in order to save one life."

So here we have another indisputable miracle. Catheter intervention beats surgery. One-third of ruptured aneurysms will rebleed. Half of all people whose aneurysms rebleed will die. Coiling up a platinum wire prevents rebleeding and saves lives.

Dr. Mangla drives the point home: "We know the benefit of coiling is real. We have seven or eight years of observation . . . Ten years ago, only 10 percent of aneurysms were coiled off with a catheter; now it is 60 percent, but in Europe it is 90 percent."

Uh-oh. "Why so much less in the United States?" I ask him, not sure I can bear hearing the answer.

"Because of the economic incentive for the surgeon," he replies.

I was afraid he'd say that. This is where modern medicine is like automotive repair: the profit incentive for a repair drives the choice of method. I wish so much that my profession were purer than that.

What I actually say out loud is, "If you chopped a hole in the side of my head and lifted my brain up instead of putting a little catheter in my artery to clog it off, I think the first thing I would do once I got off the table would be to get up and smack you."

By this point in our interview, I'm wondering what else Dr. Mangla has been doing in his corner of our medical center. Perhaps he has been doing brain transplants, and I don't know about it.

"I stent carotid arteries," he says.

Carotid stenosis is a leading cause of stroke. Stenting the artery means that Dr. Mangla doesn't need to fillet open half of the patient's head in order to strip the inside of the narrowed artery.

"Do you think you can do better than endarterectomy with surgery?" I ask.

"I do. The key to carotid stenting is experience and skill. I have done over fifty of them. Also, if I dislodge a plaque and cause a stroke, I can go up there and get it out. The surgeon cannot. Those who do cardiac work do not have the technical skill that those who do neurovascular work have. Neurovascular work is much more involved than cardiac work, and those who work in the brain have much greater technical skill. The size and tortuosity of the vessels in the neurovascular system are much more complicated."

However, Dr. Mangla goes on, "What I believe is not necessarily what the trials have said yet. So I have to give you two opinions. My opinion is that angioplasty is better, but the evidence has not yet supported it. A prospective, randomized trial that proves that angioplasty is better has not yet been done."

Fair enough, most people would say—which is true. But it also overlooks modern medicine's most important advancement: the triumph of intellectual rigor. As recently as the 1970s, it was standard practice for physicians to make decisions based solely on their own experience. In having the discipline to discount his own experience and acknowledge that what he believes and what the trials show are different, Dr. Mangla represents the height of scientific excellence. When Mangla says that the MERCI catheter and intracerebral tPA can save you from a big stroke and death, you can trust it as an evidence-based statement. Much as he might like to sell you on angioplasty for carotid stenosis as well, he won't.

Some philosophers have defined a saint as "someone able to see the world as it is, rather than what he wants it to be."

CHAPTER 8

Brain Extension

Information Technology

WELCOME, SPORTS FANS and educational experts, to morning report, which is the main teaching exercise in any residency training program. It's another beautiful morning in the hospital, and medicine fans from every level are present to witness a contest for the ages! In this corner, weighing four pounds, is the amazing Dr. Fischer's brain! And in the opposing corner, weighing less than one ounce, is a computer chip! Operating the computer will be Dr. Paul Ehrlich, chief medical informatics officer for the University Hospital of Brooklyn. Operating Dr. Fischer's brain, and all the emotional/psychological baggage every human being carries, will be Dr. Fischer.

Dr. Fischer is the undefeated champion with five Teacher of the Year Awards from three hospitals. Dr. Ehrlich will be operating the computer diagnostic program called Isabel, which is the result of 100,000 hours of clinician design and testing and contains information on 10,000 different diseases and conditions. Dr. Fischer has been a morning report teaching attending physician for 20 years, has published 10 textbooks of medicine, and has 1,000 classroom hours a year of experience. The Isabel system has been around since 2006. It is emotionless.

We are here today at information technology implementation. After decades of keeping paper records, the University Hospital of Brooklyn is finally converting to electronic ones. We are here today to see if a star teacher can be replaced with an advanced computer diagnostic and analysis system. The human and the computer will be given the same information, and 40 medical students and residents will see which system comes up with a more accurate diagnosis, treatment plan, and explanations for educational purposes. The students and residents will act as judges in a classic tale of speed, accuracy, and effectiveness!

DR. PAUL EHRLICH is investigating new programs for use in the hospital. No one doubts the benefit of an electronic system for keeping records and writing orders. Paper records are easily lost and, because of poor handwriting, can be hard to decipher. The clearest example of the superiority of electronic systems is for laboratory data. Even the best teacher will state that the ability to electronically store and retrieve lab data is an absolute necessity. The issue of using a computer program to teach and run classes for doctors is a much different story.

The stakes are high. If Paul is correct, then the concept of having a highly trained and well-read teaching/attending physician may cease to exist—any student, by accessing the Isabel system, can essentially be his or her own teaching/attending physician. Isabel was begun in 1999 after a young child's life-threatening condition was not diagnosed correctly until after the child, Isabel Maude, had developed multi-organ failure. Rather than seeking a legal course of retaliation, the child's father, Jason Maude, quit his job as a stockbroker and began developing Isabel as a computerized diagnostic system.

As reported in the May 30, 2006, issue of the *National Review of Medicine:* "Some, like Dr. Donald Berwick, president of the US-based Institute for Healthcare Improvement, still worry that physician pride is a barrier to adopting a system like ISABEL. As he told the *Boston Globe,* 'Genius diagnosticians make great stories, but they don't make great healthcare. The idea is to make accuracy reliable, not heroic.'"

Well, I certainly like the label "genius diagnosticians," but I am not so crazy about, nor do I necessarily agree with, the statement that "they don't make great healthcare." Besides my own personal clinical work, which takes up about 40 percent of my time, my professional work is based on being a genius diagnostician. Tough cases get presented to me in front of audiences of students and residents, and we dissect them together to get to the diagnosis and to learn something about the cases along the way. I am essentially a performance artist whose subject is internal medicine. A large part of my job is to get medical students and residents to be excited about medicine so that they will be inspired to learn more and work more.

This book is intended to get those same people to be overwhelmed with excitement about medicine so they feel compelled to devote their lives to a life of investigation, science, and care. The best possible outcome for me would be for ten students to choose a life of science and research and to devote their lives to the next big breakthrough. The object is to get the "best and brightest" to choose the most *difficult* problems to solve in medicine, like the cure of cancer, rather than simply the most competitive residency. The most competitive residencies are not, unfortunately, based on what is best for the future of medicine or the cure of disease. The most competitive residencies are partially based on lifestyle (fewer hours) and income. Competition is also based on the ephemeral, hard-to-measure "value" of the specialty in the eyes of the students. Twenty years ago you could not get a student to go into anesthesia or radiology. Now these are two highly competitive fields. Their "value" has gone up. Forty years ago internal medicine attracted all the best; now you are nearly begging to get even students in the top quarter of the class to go into it, and half the spots are taken by international graduates.

My goal is not attracting students into my own field. My goal is to get them, first, to take stock of everything we have learned and our great accomplishments, and get them revved up to be on the cutting edge of investigation no matter what they choose. Beyond that, I just want them to be happy. Happy that they are doing something with their lives that makes people's lives better.

Regarding Dr. Berwick's "heroic" versus "reliable" crack, I have mixed feelings. I like heroism for me personally but not for the health care system. For the system to function well, a calm reliability is infinitely superior to dramatic, heroic diagnostics. On a routine flight from New York to Los Angeles, I don't want heroics from the airplane pilot; I want calm, dependable reliability. The same is true of medicine. Unfortunately, you can't depend on a doctor's heroic qualities coming to the fore, but you can pretty much rely on his or her weaknesses always being there. We therefore need a safe, reliable electronic system that can detect and correct mistakes. We can still keep a couple of guys like me around for "medical entertainment," but we can't run a hospital based on our heroic accuracy.

Throughout this book I describe "miracles" that are becoming "routine," but if you think I advocate miracles for the vast majority of care, you would be wrong. Reliability and reproducibility are the ways to go. A fact-based, evidence-based system of routine tests and procedures must be in place for the majority of diagnoses. The concept of private practice—which is that individual doctors can do and order whatever they see fit, with the only check on the system being the doctor's own personal integrity and knowledge—will fade. I don't mean that we have to do away with the human side of warmth, kindness, and empathy. I mean that we can routinize certain aspects of medicine that will really help people: vaccinations, blood pressure control, diabetes management, cholesterol control.

Even in the high-tech arena of the hospital, the current system is based on human memory: the doctor has to remember to order those blood tests, then remember to check the results, and then remember to implement therapy. Now, I am essentially a human memory expert. My entire day is spent in front of trainees getting them to learn enormous amounts of data. I have all sorts of games, songs, toys, and tricks to enhance memory. And physicians should, absolutely, have a strong memory that taps into a vast well of knowledge. However, I also believe that, in an improved system, a sole reliance on human memory will go the way of the eight-track tape player and the rotary phone. Standard tests should be automatically checked and therapy automatically recommended, with the physician there to provide human warmth and modifications in case the patient's conditions don't fall into the usual algorithms.

Private and attending physicians often become upset with my message. One of their concerns is liability. Right now, attending physicians of record take upon themselves all the burden of liability. Removing decision-making capacity without altering liability would be akin to taxation without representation. However, an automated system of checks and balances will inherently result in a marked decrease in mistakes, and with that decrease will come a marked decrease in the potential for liability. Besides that, it is time for the profession to come to the realization that establishing a system for the best possible result for the patient has got to be our number one goal. An airplane pilot might feel that there is a diminishment in his personal glory when a computer flies the plane and when air traffic control guides the flight plan and timing, but glory must give way to safety.

I do not think that doctors will be able to self-police. We couldn't bring ourselves to limit duty hours for residents; the change had to be forced on us. We couldn't bring ourselves to fight effectively for health care finance reform in the 1990s; that battle is being fought by people outside the medical profession. We have not always been able to change institutional procedures from within. For example, at one point in our emergency department, it became clear that we were not getting our patients with myocardial infarctions the angioplasty they needed within the mandated 90 minutes of coming to the door. The system in place was as follows: the emergency doctor notified the cardiology fellow, the fellow talked to the general cardiologist, the general cardiologist notified the invasive cardiologist, and the invasive cardiologist notified the laboratory. It took two and a half hours to get the balloon into the patient's obstructed artery. The head of the invasive laboratory was asked over and over to change the system. The institution's president finally had to say to him: "Change the system or you're fired." Now the emergency department physician makes simultaneous notifications. Since that change in the system, nearly every single emergency angioplasty has happened within 90 minutes. Change may have to be forced on us if we cannot police ourselves to get the automated, reliable system of double checking that we need.

PATIENTS MAY BE one of the drivers of change. Minky Worden is the media director for the nonprofit organization Human Rights Watch; we have a chance meeting one day that turns into an informal interview about medical informatics.

Minky says, "I dumped my last doctor because he didn't have an electronic medical record. I figured that anyone these days who does not have an electronic record can't be at the cutting edge of his work. I don't want someone stuck in the past. For me, an electronic record means you know what you are doing and you are trying to be the best. Besides, I don't want some guy with a paper record who is fumbling around trying to find things. I want someone with automated systems. So I left that doctor and got one who is more advanced from my point of view."

Minky is not in health care. She is one of the myriad ordinary educated people in New York. But her words have a striking effect on me. They indicate that people are now so interested in medical informatics that they will actually base their choice of a physician on whether he or she embraces this state of the art in health care. This is a very important development. Patient awareness will accelerate the speed at which information technology is adopted, because nothing affects a private practitioner more than the ability to be competitive in the marketplace, particularly in a doctor-dense area like New York City.

Minky Worden's husband, L. Gordon Crovitz, also takes part in the discussion. He says, "I would think you guys would want everything put in an electronic database because of the outstanding research possibilities. If all the patients in the country have their data in the same electronic database, it would seem to me that you could ask all kinds of interesting research questions and solve all sorts of problems. Wouldn't this advantage be obvious to everybody? Think about all the clinical trials and individual enrollments in research you could avoid by having everybody's information available to you on every disease. Wouldn't this be more efficient? I mean, if I were a patient, I wouldn't mind having the data there anonymously available for investigation purposes. Think about how you could advance medicine."

He happens to be totally right. Since he has the late-forties, balding, graying, high-intelligence look of a deep guy, I hazard a guess that he is a computer geek.

Not exactly, he replies. He is a journalist. For 27 years, Gordon worked at the *Wall Street Journal* and was the publisher from 2006 to 2007, essentially guiding the content and direction of the whole paper, as well as the executive vice president of Dow Jones. In other words, he has nothing to do with medicine or information technology in hospitals. He falls in the category of generally smart and well-informed guy.

Gordon goes on: "Think about all the unnecessary tests you could avoid. You wouldn't have to have your CT scan or MRI repeated every time you entered a new hospital or doctor's office. You wouldn't have to have all your blood tests repeated. If you went into the hospital with an emergency, all your information would be readily accessible. Wouldn't this be safer and more intelligent?"

Gordon has the easy, pleasant conversational tone of a guy just asking an intelligent question. So, it is probably inappropriate for me to tell him to "mind your place, Gordy! I am the expert doctor here! We don't need an 'outsider' telling us what to do. Just shut up and eat your chicken!" So instead I say, "Well, there would be a lot of confidentiality issues to overcome. We are very sensitive to those violations. And besides that, you have to enter patients for research prospectively, asking individual questions."

Gordon persists, not because he is trying to be difficult, but because he has thought this through: "Then people can sign consent to have their data unlinked from their names for confidential research purposes. I would sign up for that. The point is not to let the information be wasted. The point is to try to understand things better. I bet there are a lot of interesting questions you can ask and answer from a huge database like that."

I am impressed. Gordon Crovitz is engaging in a logical, persuasive, rational argument in the service of advancing medical knowledge. It is hard to disagree with him, especially because he is right. Information technology and communication in health care are about 15 to 20 years behind the financial industry. It's not safe, but it is private. There is nothing so private and confidential as a paper record that the doctor can't even find.

Now both Gordon and Minky pop in. We talk about why you can have your entire financial history on a tiny chip in your credit card that allows you to go anywhere in the world and have your entire financial history available at the swipe of a card, but if you are going to the hospital, there is no information.

I look to the right.

"Yeah, you can have a little chip with all your information on a card. That way all your medications and tests are readily available," says Minky.

I look left.

"Your EKG and all your allergies will be on the card, so that if you go to the emergency room unconscious, they will know how to treat you and they won't give you a medicine you are allergic to," says Gordon.

My head spins right again.

"You could have a chip in your forearm implanted with all your data, including the actual images of your X-rays. When you enter the hospital, all they have to do is scan your arm and pick up the data. I would sign up for that right now," says Minky.

They've got me surrounded! I am boxed in by a pair of rational, intelligent New Yorkers. My mind is being batted back and forth like a tennis ball across a net.

But they are both correct. I become embarrassed for my profession. Why aren't we doctors leading the effort on this? Is this what it's come to? We have to wait for the general public to pull us by the ear to do the right thing? In New York there are 44 hospitals. There are no routine links in information between them. I can go to a cash machine anywhere in the world and access all my information and money in a second. If I go even so much as across the street from my hospital, it is as if I didn't even exist. If you are brought to an emergency room unconscious, you'd better hope they don't give you a medication you are allergic to. They have no way of knowing, and you may die. Physicians have not fixed this. So the next time someone in health care gives you the "We need to maintain our autonomy" argument or the "We know what we are doing" argument, you must do as Gordon Crovitz did to me: just point out the facts and explore the possibilities.

Minky's actions were even louder than her words. In essence, she told her former doctor, "As soon as you get into the twenty-first century, you can call me. Meanwhile I am going down the street."

WE ARE BACK at morning report. I am about to enter into my contest of man versus machine. I will analyze a case at the same time that Isabel, the electronic database, tries to analyze it. I am confident that I will prevail: there is no way some readily accessible computer database is more accurate than my brain! I am also much more entertaining, and cuter—my students love me! I'm not afraid. No sir, not me. That's probably why I have never so much as once tried to even test a computerized diagnostic system. Plus, the six-figure salary I earn for working 8 to 12 hours a day is probably more cost-effective than this system, which is available for only, uh, 24 hours a day and can be implemented for, uh, oops, $35,000.

Anyway, on to the test! The case is presented. Dr. Paul Ehrlich enters the data, and I do the traditional case dissection with all my best methods of teaching.

It turns out I am a little faster than the Isabel system. It turns out that my list of diagnoses is similar to Isabel's. Who wins? Honestly, seriously, I think it is too soon to tell. I breathe a huge sigh of relief that the Isabel system does not actually come up with anything that I missed. It does, however, come up with some stuff that is not relevant to the case. For now, the contest ends in a draw, with a slight edge going to the human.

However, this is not a fair or accurate assessment for ordinary decision making. In the test this morning, we were comparing Isabel against me, an extremely well-prepared teacher. In real-life circumstances, Isabel's results would be compared with those of a much newer physician with a much smaller knowledge base who is much less well read than I am. Also, there is a big difference between analyzing a case at an educational conference and the real-life situation of evaluating your patient at three in the morning.

What I provide in teaching is more than just the facts. My manner, style, and emotions can enhance students' retention of the material. I provide the drama that makes the process considerably more engaging.

Dr. Paul Ehrlich is responsible for implementing the electronic medical record at the University Hospital of Brooklyn. He is also the man who brings Isabel into morning report. Because he is an M.D., he will be heard with greater ease by the clinical staff than he would be otherwise. Because he comes to morning report with regularity, he will have a greater chance at changing behavior than an outsider would have. His job is to see if Isabel will be a useful evaluation tool for physicians in their routine care of patients.

His job is to see if Isabel is better than me. Paul is one of my greatest friends and allies at the hospital. He simply wants things to run better. He has a huge job. It is not just that he has to choose and design the right systems; he also has to change physician behavior—and that, my friends, is a difficult thing to do. What does it matter if he puts the right systems in place if no one uses them? He also has to catch their attention to get them to learn how to use them. This is a little like being a dentist for a lion with a toothache. The lion needs you and is suffering, but you don't want to be the one to have to put your hands in the lion's mouth.

Paul is an obstetrician-gynecologist. He is also an active patient. Paul developed some very serious orthopedic problems with the bones in his wrist that made it difficult for him to operate, which is significant, since gynecology is a surgical specialty. As a result of his wrist injury, Paul retooled to be an informatics specialist. He could have just sat on the sidelines of life, subsisting on disability. Paul is in his midforties, chunky and jolly, with a goatee and glasses, a quick wit, and a tendency toward biting sarcasm that makes him one of my favorite characters. He is also the grandson of two concentration camp survivors, and this tends to give him a long view on history.

"The amount of data that a physician is required to have readily available at this point in time, given all of the explosions we have had, is beyond the capacity of the average human to attain, it really is," Paul says. "If you go back about twenty years, an Eastern European Jewish woman who was pregnant needed to be tested for a single genetic disease, Tay-Sachs. That was it. Now for the general pregnant woman, we are up to something like 15 diseases. The average physician is challenged to remember them all. He has diagnostic information, therapeutic information.

"Now start multiplying the number of classes of drugs by the number of drugs in each class. Well, there are over six thousand drugs in the U.S. pharmacopeia. So the amount of information that is required for the good practice of medicine is beyond the capacity of the average physician, and even for your above-average clinician. That is one major obstacle. The other major obstacle is that historically in medicine we have taken a very Aristotelian approach to the way we think. That is, we think that if we can understand the mechanism of how things work, then we can reason how to correct them.

"The problem is that there are often those paradoxical responses. From an Aristotelian perspective, a classic one is 'Don't give beta-blockers to someone with congestive heart failure; you are going to decrease the contractility of the heart and thereby worsen the patient's condition.' Now along comes something called evidence-based medicine, in which the empiric question is put to the test, and your null hypothesis is defeated. In this case you end up with an even greater amount of knowledge that you need to retain. You now cannot even simply reason your way through everything. There have been studies and meta-analysis and randomized clinical trials that say: 'Your approach is intuitively correct, but the practice is incorrect.' So how do you support the intuition, the clinical judgment, and the technical skill of clinicians so that they can continue to practice medicine in an ever-exploding environment of new discoveries? How do you keep them current, keep them safe, and help advance patient care?

"I think that is where technology plays a role. Technology is a tool. Properly used, it is a tool. Improperly used, it is a toy.

"Access to information starts with an electronic medical record. Remember that every patient has a single medical history but multiple medical charts. Patients see an internist, and they see an ophthalmologist, and they see their dermatologist and gynecologist. So if the doctors are not part of the same multispecialty group, the patients have fragmented charts. Patients are not reliable historians. They say, 'I am taking a water pill from Doctor A, and other is a white pill from Doctor B, and the other is a blue pill from Doctor C,' but they can't understand and don't accurately remember what they are on and why, so the care remains fragmented."

I ask Paul about the role of the teacher and the "heroic diagnostician" in analysis of patient care. To be precise, I ask: "Is there really any added value in having a Conrad Fischer there to analyze the case, or can you just have anybody sitting there going into a database and dissecting the case with Isabel?"

He responds, "The answer is two things: there is an art and there is a science. You have immense recall of scientific fact, as does Isabel. The difference is that you have a unique mechanism of parlaying that knowledge into retainable information for other people in the room.

"The problems we are confronting are different. There is no central repository of information. This is especially true in pharmacy. My eighty-five-year-old father has to buy some of his medications in pharmacies in Canada. There is no communication. So having a central database is critical. One of the projects we are involved in right now is NYCLIX, the New York Clinical Information Exchange."

Now Paul gets all geeky on me. As a manly man, Paul always likes to point out that there is a difference between a nerd and a geek. Nerds hide out from life after having spent too much time with video games in the basement of their mother's house. Nerdism is a mild version of social anxiety disorder and agoraphobia. Geeks are technoheads who spend a million hours on the computer designing new systems. Geeks are more like artists and creators than nerds are.

So my favorite geek whips around his computer screen and says, "Want to see?" In an instant, we are looking at the entry portal for the NYCLIX system.

"This is the beginning of having the hospitals communicate with each other," Paul says.

"So this is like Columbus crossing the Atlantic in 1492?" I ask.

"To some extent, yes. Right now, Downstate has a server that only has Downstate information on it. New York University has a server that only has that institution's on it. Now when a patient comes to the emergency department, a query is sent to the fourteen hospitals in the five boroughs to see what information is available on that patient, but the patient has to opt in on it. This is not Big Brother—you have to directly consent for it—but this is the first-ever electronic consortium between hospitals in New York City. There has never been as many as fourteen hospitals involved in data sharing. But it means you can get a patient's lab data, EKGs, and all the other tests he or she has had."

"So this is like having the first transatlantic cable laid down?"

"Sort of," Paul responds. "It works on a federated model, but it can work together like it is almost seamless."

"It's amazing that it has taken until the year 2008 to do something like this. So, Paul, where do we go from here?"

"The Department of Health in New York State is giving grants to implement this. Each of the hospitals is also contributing some money. We joined about a year ago." Then he says something that drives me crazy with its irrational, short-sighted illogic: "Honestly, we are not sure that NYCLIX is going to survive, because there is no sustainable business model for it yet."

Where is Gordon Crovitz? Where is my *Wall Street Journal* guy to slap some sense into the entire system? Apparently that is what we need: a business-oriented person to get us to do the right thing. Hurry up! I can see Minky Worden reaching for her bag walking out the door headed for, say, New Jersey. "Thank you, New York," she says. "If you can't get this electronic system up and working, I will go elsewhere for care until you can prove to me you are using state-of-the-art technology."

But then I recall that it is not any better in New Jersey. Minky is now like the heroine in a silent movie. An unseen fiend cackles, "Ha, ha, ha! My dear, you are trapped! There is nowhere to run!" The poor damsel lies tied to a railroad track awaiting the oncoming train of her own illnesses.

PART 3

Giving and Receiving "Thanks!"

CHAPTER 9

Cured

Cardiology Patients Offer Heartfelt Gratitude

MONIQUE KEARNEY IS an elementary school teacher. She is a quiet, somewhat introverted person who sits calmly on the edge of the examining table and tells me, "The symptoms were keeping me from my life."

Her tone is not angry, frustrated, or frightened. At first I wonder if it was really all that bad.

Then she continues: "I couldn't do anything. I couldn't breathe. I was tired all the time. I couldn't get up a flight of stairs. Even when these symptoms weren't occurring, it was weird and disconcerting. You go about things that you need to do as best as you can, but everything is more of a burden because you are tired all the time . . . I went through my whole pregnancy with atrial fibrillation last year. It was very hard."

The left atrium is the small chamber in the heart that contracts to pass blood into the left ventricle, which passes the blood to the rest of the body. Ordinarily, when the atrium contracts, it pushes only 10 to 20 percent of the blood that makes up the total cardiac output. But the loss of atrial contraction can decrease cardiac output by 30 to 50 percent. This is why Ms. Kearney felt tired, weak, and short of breath. Why did she get worse with pregnancy? A normal person has about five liters of blood volume. Blood volume goes up by one to two liters with pregnancy. That is why her symptoms got so much worse.

The chambers of the heart are supposed to contract in a nice, smooth, top-to-bottom flow of electrical activity that squeezes blood up and out of the heart into the aorta. When atrial fibrillation (AFib) occurs, there is no organized electrical activity of the heart. Blood pools in the heart, and that stasis can form clots. These clots may fly to the brain and cause a stroke, so physicians prescribe the blood thinner called warfarin. It is a pain-in-the-ass medication that needs to be monitored with blood testing. The international normalized ratio (INR) has to be maintained at two to three times the normal rate of blood clotting. If the INR is too low, you clot. If it is too high, you bleed. I hope that in 20 years we will look back at the possible danger of this medication as ridiculously primitive. But for now, blood testing is not as difficult as having a clot and a stroke.

From the 1960s to the late 1990s, we used medicines and electricity to try to convert the heart from atrial fibrillation to a normal heart rhythm. For 30 years, we shocked and prodded and drugged. It took us three decades to realize that the successful conversion rate after using every intervention was about 7 percent after a year. It turns out that about 7 percent of patients will spontaneously convert their AFib to sinus (normal) rhythm after a year. In other words, all our intervention did not make a difference in the ultimate outcome. We quit trying to convert AFibtosinus.

When the paddles of the electrical cardioversion machines were developed, it seemed logical to shock AFib into sinus rhythm. But if the heart is abnormally shaped because of high blood pressure, then shocking someone does not work, because it does not change the shape of the heart. Even if you get the patient temporarily into normal sinus rhythm, his or her heart will eventually pop back into AFib. Nobody realized this until researchers actually studied arrhythmia-converting methods in the 1990s. It wasn't the danger of the investigation that made us fail to study it earlier; rather, it was the certainty that we already knew what would happen.

In other words: the therapies resulted in a contracting atrium. A contracting atrium is good. Would you withhold therapy from an ill person just to prove the treatment works?

AFib management at the end of the 20th century represented a failure to apply the scientific method. For us, now, to begin widespread use of a new treatment without a clinical trial would be dangerous and unethical. For a cardiologist in the 1960s, it would have been equally unethical to withhold a treatment all physicians believed was effective. Some physicians have called me a traitor for talking too much about such failures. They say I am damaging the profession. They miss my point: I am being honest and open because I want people to know they can trust the medical profession—that if we make a mistake, we will study it, find the truth, admit we were wrong, and try to fix it. The routine attempt to convert AFib was for 30 years a huge professional and scientific failure. Studying it was an enormous triumph of professionalism and integrity. Options come to open minds, and with options come hopes.

Ms. Kearney had an unusual type of AFib. She needed a physician with an open mind and an investigational approach. Dr. John Kassotis is a rare man. He has an M.D. and a Ph.D. After his three-year residency for internal medicine, he did three years of a fellowship in cardiology, followed by an additional two years to sub-subspecialize in electrophysiology (EP). He also earned a Ph.D. in physiology, for a grand total of 15 years of school and training after college to be able to place a catheter into the center of a beating human heart and map the intricacies of cardiac conduction. He can insert a pacemaker to speed up a heart so that the patient doesn't pass out. He places implantable cardioverter defibrillators that shock stopped hearts back to life. He routinely works in measurements of timing at the level of 1/100th of a second. The slightest mistake, and someone's life will be cut short.

In the dozen trips I make to see John and his partner, Adam Budzikowski (who also has two doctorates), they are as constant as the sun. Available, clear, logical, matter of fact, calm. John Kassotis routinely tells patients, "I am an electrician." In fact, he and Adam radiate knowledge and wear the aura of expertise. I can just imagine the ads for their fragrance: they are wearing Calvin Klein's newest scent, Intelligence. Cutting-edge change is a routine part of their work.

"When did this new device get approved?" I ask Adam.

"Monday."

"When did you put in your first one?"

"Tuesday."

Ms. Kearney's AFib was not from high blood pressure, leaky valves, or an abnormally shaped heart. Instead electrophysiologic testing showed that it came from an abnormality in the conduction system of her heart. Given this discovery, Dr. Kassotis decided to attempt to eliminate the source of her AFib through ablation. (The verb *ablate* simply means "remove"; another synonym for it is *kill*. Like members of the Mafia or the CIA, we doctors don't like to use words as crass or direct as *kill*. Instead of *neutralize* or *whack,* we say *ablate*.) He put a catheter into the right side of her heart, where the pulmonary veins drain into the organ, and heated the tip with radiofrequency electrical waves. The idea was to fry the source of the arrhythmia, in a procedure a bit like electrolysis or laser hair removal for the heart.

We don't throw that word *cure* around too much in medicine. We are, as a profession, a little like the lover who won't say "I love you." Maybe it won't last? Maybe it will go away? Maybe I will disappoint you. Yet, content-packed four-letter words like *cure* and *love* are exactly what life is about. I want to hear Dr. Kassotis say that Ms. Kearney is cured. Instead he tells me, "Ms. Kearney has been successfully ablated, but she might need a repeat procedure." I wonder if, afterward, he felt the same excitement inside that I felt exploding in me when I heard about this procedure. But after his day's work, all John Kassotis did was send a two-line message to his chief of medicine: "Young female with lone atrial fibrillation since age 31. Successfully ablated to normal sinus rhythm. The first complete four vein isolation restoring sinus rhythm."

He gave it two lines and a shrug. Had his boss not passed the note on to me, I might never have known. In the hundreds of interviews I conducted for this book, the physicians rarely expressed gratitude for all the good they are able to do. Similarly, they seemed to have no idea how to accept gratitude from their patients. Time and again I spoke with patients who were amazed by what their doctors were able to do, and their physicians never seemed to get it.

Ms. Kearney had instant relief of her symptoms after the procedure.

"In the next hour I felt better," she says. "I knew that if this procedure did not work for me, I would not have any other options. I would just have to live with it."

A month after our original interview, I call Ms. Kearney to see how it is going. I hear children in the background; she is clearly at the playground.

"I still get some palpitations, but there is no more atrial fibrillation. I am doing okay, though. I am pregnant, and I am doing okay."

For the doctor, it is routine; for the patient, it is a miracle, options are found amidst the hopelessness.

MS. FAUSTINA SKINNER didn't seem to have any options, any hope, anything to be grateful for.

"I used to be in a bad mood all the time," she says. "I didn't have any energy, and I was upset with everyone. I was really difficult to deal with. I wasn't good to be around."

It never occurred to her that things could be otherwise. In our interview, Ms. Skinner is accompanied by her home health aide. She is a 68-year-old woman from Jamaica. Every time Ms. Skinner talks about how short-tempered she was, the home health aide smiles or laughs because, today, Ms. Skinner is a happy woman. She is cheerful, talkative, and relaxed. Like most of the other patients I interviewed for this book, she is happy to talk about her medical past. In the age of reality television, talking about your private life is routine, and only 2 percent of the patients I speak to don't want me to use their real names. They all want to tell their stories.

Ms. Skinner was always in a bad mood because she could barely move or walk. Her heart did not pump efficiently, despite the best medical therapy.

"I could only make it about three steps before I got short of breath," she says. "I couldn't even make it to the bathroom. I would get winded. Sometimes I could not even turn over in bed without getting short of breath."

Ms. Skinner suffered from a low ejection fraction. Furthermore, her atrium and ventricle were not passing the blood between each other efficiently. It was like a relay race in which the runner does not show up in time for the next runner to get moving. *Yo, atrium! Where are you? Where's the blood? Aw, forget it! I'm going to contract anyway, even if I am only half full.*

Ms. Skinner was already taking medications for her illness. In the past, the only remaining option would have been a heart transplant. But a new technology called a biventricular pacemaker has become available. It helps pump blood in the right direction. With her biventricular pacemaker, Ms. Skinner can suddenly do things inconceivable to her a few weeks ago, like walking six or seven blocks without stopping.

"I only stop for red lights now," she says. "I can do what I want."

A little old lady with heart failure is, almost overnight, walking more than the average healthy American. Dr. Budzikowski and Dr. Kassotis had told me that patients with biventricular pacemakers saw enormous improvements in their tolerance for exercise. They told me that housebound patients were able to walk out of their homes for the first time in months or years. But even an over-the-top optimist like me had not expected the results to be as dramatic as Ms. Skinner's.

"I feel happier," she says. "My mood is better. I am not so short-tempered. I am easier to be around. I am easier to deal with. I have energy, and I don't feel so helpless."

I say, "The next thing you will tell me is that you want to go dancing."

"I did go dancing!" She and the home health aide start laughing. "I started moving right away, so I started moving with the music. I can go dancing."

"Well, then, next you'll want me to get a man for you."

She and her aide start laughing again.

A pacemaker as a treatment for depression. And a prerequisite for dancing. I am happy and done. I start to leave.

"One last thing, Doc."

"Yes, Ms. Skinner?"

"Can't you write me a prescription for that man?"

ROBERT KANE, A 50-year-old man in the prime of his life, couldn't walk two blocks and couldn't breathe when he climbed stairs. He had severe congestive heart failure, and he was not getting better with medications. With no correctable cause and no clogged arteries to bypass, Robert was facing either a heart transplant or death. It would most likely be a sudden death.

Robert had been diagnosed with idiopathic cardiomyopathy, which in translation means, "Your heart is weak, and we don't know why. It might have been weakened by a virus. We do know that you will shortly die." In his case, the normal ejection fraction (the percentage of blood pumped out of the left ventricle with each heartbeat) of 60 to 75 percent had been reduced to 10 percent. To improve it, he had a defibrillator attached to his chest.

He tells me about that experience: "One night it picked up an abnormal rhythm and gave me a shock that sent me across the room. Another time I was standing in a store, and the device detected an abnormality. It started to talk—the device, I mean. It said, 'Abnormal rhythm detected.

Please stand clear. Prepare for shock.' It was embarrassing. I was at the checkout line in a store. I started to walk out. I felt like the Bionic Man. No shock came, but it was very frightening."

Dr. Adam Budzikowski placed a combined biventricular pacemaker and implantable defibrillator into Robert.

"I'm feeling good about life now," Robert says. "It is tough knowing you have this wire in your heart, but I can walk without getting short of breath now . . . I haven't had any shocks. I feel better. I can walk more, I can climb stairs, I feel normal. But every step to me is precious."

Dr. Budzikowski explains: "The biventricular pacemaker resynchronizes Robert's heart. It makes all the chambers beat together the way they are supposed to. Blood comes out more efficiently. It doesn't cure him. But it will buy him five more years, at least, from having to have a transplant."

I am sitting with Dr. Budzikowski in his office, which is wallpapered with pictures of his daughter. On a huge computer console he shows me a three-dimensional image of a heart and the areas of good and bad conduction. He is rotating the image in a way unimaginable more than five years ago. He shows me exactly where he ablated the tissue in Robert's heart using a radiofrequency catheter with an irrigated tip. Cool!

Adam Budzikowski, the electrophysiologist, enters the beating human heart as a matter of routine. A pacer here. A defibrillator there. Here a shock, there a shock, everywhere a cath, cath. Old MacDonald had an EP lab. The 1950s saw the invention of the heart-lung bypass machine, which allowed open heart surgery. Dr. Budzikowski is a pioneer in the next wave of cardiac repair. Without cracking the chest open, he enters the heart with a catheter and repairs the conduction system. He pierces the septum (the wall between the right and left atria) to do his work. He does this without exposing patients to the risks of bypass surgery, which include infection and brain damage. The big thing in the future of procedures lies in small. Smaller incisions. Shorter recovery time. Shorter hospital stays.

With a device that did not exist even three years ago, Dr. Budzikowski was able to snatch Robert Kane from a heart transplant or sudden death. The biventricular pacemaker has eliminated virtually all of Robert's shortness of breath. It won't last, but when you are on death row waiting for your name to be called, the defibrillator is like the governor staying your sentence. With the biventricular pacemaker relieving your symptoms, it is like the governor also giving you permission to wait at home with your family.

Dr. Budzikowski says, "We bought Robert Kane five more years, but it is not a cure."

Robert Kane says, "I am just grateful to God and to Dr. Bud for giving me five more years of feeling good and to watch my daughter grow up."

Speaking to Robert on the phone, I hear the strength of responsible fatherhood in his voice. In the background I hear one child squeezing through piano lessons, another talking to Mommy. I smell love in the air.

AINSLEY HARRIS IS in his late sixties. He is sitting in a patient care room wearing a baseball cap that says "Walk with Jesus. Exercise your faith." He exudes a calm decency and politeness.

"I was having symptoms of skipped beats and palpitations every once in a while for about the last three years. They didn't bother me that much, and I did not have any big symptoms. One night last year I got up in the middle of the night to go to the bathroom. I didn't make it. I fell to the ground . . . I died."

Mr. Harris's wife, Adelia, a retired head nurse from a cardiac care unit, started to do CPR on him.

"I called the ambulance, and they were there in minutes," she says. "When the ambulance arrived, the monitor showed ventricular tachycardia, although I thought I saw ventricular fibrillation too."

Ventricular tachycardia presents itself in many different ways. You can have it for just a few beats and feel nothing. You can have it for longer and feel palpitations or signs of decreased cardiac output such as lightheadedness, low blood pressure, chest pain, or shortness of breath. Or it can kill you.

"When I think of it now, I know I was dead for a while," Mr. Harris says.

The Harrises have a little argument about how long he was dead. This is amusing in a certain way.

Ainsley Harris had an implantable defibrillator put in. This, by itself, was not a big breakthrough. Implantable defibrillators have been around for years. They shock the heart muscle when it is in distress. The defibrillator records the heart's rhythm at the time of the shock. Mr. Harris was shocked each time he was in ventricular tachycardia (V-tach).

"What do the shocks feel like? Is it like being punched in the chest?"

"It is much worse than being punched . . . It is like being executed. It is like you are in the electric chair, and they are executing you."

Then one night it was different. Mr. Harris started to get shock after shock.

Mrs. Harris says, "At first I thought the device might be defective, but when I looked at the tracing of the rhythm later, they were all legitimate. He had V-tach every time."

"How many times did it happen?"

"Twelve times. All legitimate."

I try to imagine what it must be like to have the simulated experience of being executed 12 times.

Dr. Adam Budzikowski comes into the room. "First we ablated his atrial flutter," he says, "but we could still induce V-tach, so we tried something new. The implantable defibrillator was in 'storm'—that means a flurry of shocks for repeated episodes of V-tach. We did the first ablation of ventricular tachycardia with an irrigated catheter tip. This puts cool water out of the tip so it does not overheat the surrounding tissue and damage normal heart muscle. This is the way to melt the electrograms."

"What's an electrogram?"

"It is the electrical source of the arrhythmia in the heart muscle."

Dr. Budzikowski shows me the image of Mr. Harris's heart on his computer. The computer-generated colors tell which tissue is normal and which is not. "You see here," he says, pointing to an area in gray, indicating dead tissue. "This is the source of the arrhythmia. We melted the electrograms surrounding this area so that the V-tach could not spread."

I ask what this means.

"It means he is cured."

Finally, someone has used one of my favorite words.

I go back to Ainsley Harris. He confirms that since the procedure several months earlier, he has not had an episode of ventricular tachycardia. He has not had a single additional shock. He feels normal. No palpitations. No shocks.

No dying.

Then he surprises me.

"You know what gives me hope?" he says. "It makes me happy to know there will be other options later. I know that the technology continues to get better and better, so I know that other new things will come that can help me in the future."

Here is a man who wears his faith on his baseball cap.

He says to me, "I was like Lazarus raised from the dead. You know who that makes Dr. Bud, don't you?"

Time and time again, I heard similar expressions of enormous gratitude from patients. Even for things they could have gotten from any competent doctor, not just superstars like Dr. Kassotis and Dr. Budzikowski, people felt a deep sense of appreciation. But I never detected much absorption of this feeling on the part of the physician. What is the emotional defect on the part of physicians that they do not seem to feel it? Is this why they convey to students their sense of dissatisfaction? There seems to be an emotional hole in the heart of the medical profession. It is not a lack of compassion or caring on the part of the physician, but rather the physician's own inability to accept thanks. Maybe if dissatisfied physicians could feel this gratitude, they would feel more fulfilled by their calling. Perhaps if they felt appreciated, they would feel better paid. If they felt appreciated and well paid, maybe they would believe that now is the best time ever to be practicing medicine, because we are able to do so much more than ever before.

Chest pain relieved. Heart attacks interrupted. Biventricular pacemakers put in that take a patient dancing for the first time in years. Rhythm disorders ablated and cured. There is a lot to feel grateful about in medicine, both for the patient and the caregiver who has more power than ever before to cure disease. Gratitude can be fuel for the medical profession, if only most physicians could feel it. It might inspire our best minds to find the next new device. We need to develop the next biventricular pacemaker, to advance stem cell research to find new ways to create organs for transplant, and to find immunosuppressive drugs that allow the recipient to tolerate a donated organ without side effects. Because we need to know what to do when Robert Kane's five years are up.

*If science can definitely prove that something the Buddha says
was wrong, then go with the science.*   —Dalai Lama

CHAPTER 10

You Sexy Thing

The Everyday Miracles of Evidence-Based Medicine

DR. JASON LAZAR HAS a Groucho Marx mustache perched on a face that likes to smile.

"I guess the stuff I do in noninvasive cardiology does not have the kind of sexiness you are looking for," he tells me in all seriousness. "I know it is not as dramatic as the stuff the other guys do. People don't think about how terrific the prescription is that we wrote for them. "

Jason is the director of noninvasive cardiology at SUNY Downstate, and he looks sad and disappointed. I hate it when Jason looks sad, because Jason is a funny guy. He has the most toys in the building. He is also a great teacher, and I love great teachers.

The most common reason for hospital admission in the United States is congestive heart failure, a weakening of the heart muscle usually caused by a heart attack. Virtually every patient diagnosed with congestive heart failure gets an echocardiogram. With echocardiography we can detect through sound the precise movements of the heart, every twitch of the cardiac wall, and every subtle movement of the valves.

Jason runs stress testing and echocardiography, one of the most important areas of the hospital. You need an extra fellowship just to read an echocardiogram the way Jason does.

I press him to tell me about what is new in his area.

"I know you are talking to the guys who do angioplasty and pop open arteries and the guys who put in defibrillators," he replies. "What I do doesn't get noticed as easily."

He is enormously skilled and experienced, but he tells me his job is exciting as a plumber's: you don't notice the plumbing when it works, but when it is backed up it catches your attention.

He goes on. "I mean, there is the case of the person with the patent foramen ovale we closed, but I know you want more."

Excuse me? A foramen ovale is a hole in the embryonic heart. More specifically, it is an opening between the two atrial chambers that allows the flow of blood in the heart to bypass the lungs. It is supposed to close at birth, so that the blood will go into the lungs. In cases where it doesn't close, it is called a patent (open) foramen ovale (PFO).

"What do you mean, closed a PFO?"

"Well, we had a patient who was short of breath and had her PFO closed with a catheter, and she stopped being short of breath."

I call this patient. She says, "I was so short of breath I could barely move. They put a catheter in my heart and put in a device that closed the hole."

I ask if the improvement was dramatic.

"No, not really," she says.

I say, "Oh, that's too bad. What happened?"

"Well," she replies, "I did start to be able to walk normally, and I did stop having to use half my medications, and I did start to feel normal, and I did start to be able to walk up stairs for the first time in years. I did have a hole in my heart, and they closed it."

What is wrong with these people? Here is a person who gets one of the most advanced procedures on the planet without a surgeon having to saw through her chest. Her life has changed dramatically, and both she and her doctor are acting as if they just did the dishes.

She continues, "Well, I did get short of breath in the middle of the night and I did not know I had a hole in my heart until Dr. Lazarus told me."

I ponder her slip of the tongue in changing Jason Lazar's name to Lazarus, brought back from the dead.

For hundreds of years we have known about the diagnosis of congestive heart failure, but nothing effective to do about it until recently. In fact, the most common medication from the 18th century to the early 1980s, digoxin (also known as digitalis), turned out to be toxic when combined with another medication for alleviating symptoms. Digoxin works on the heart in a way that's like smacking the heart with a stick to make it work harder. It wasn't until the early 1980s, centuries after congestive heart failure was first identified, that someone had this radical idea: decrease the amount of work the heart must do.

Angiotensin converting enzyme (ACE) inhibitors open up the arteries in front of the heart so that more blood comes out with each beat. This means less work for the heart. Less work means less oxygen is consumed. Less oxygen consumed means less likelihood of a myocardial infarction and arrhythmia. ACE inhibitors are the first medications that were proven to lower mortality in patients with congestive heart failure. For every 100 people put on an ACE inhibitor, the risk of death goes down by about 25 percent. There is about a 20 percent risk of death each year for people with congestive heart failure. Thus, the use of ACE inhibitors translates to a 5 percent absolute reduction in the risk of death each year. That means you only need to put 20 people with congestive heart failure on an ACE inhibitor to save 1 life. Who says there's no drama here?

The first ACE inhibitor, captopril, was approved in 1981, which in the context of this book is ancient history. The real breakthrough came in the late 1990s. Amazingly, the medication had been right under our noses since the 1950s. Since then, medications known as beta-blockers have been used to lower blood pressure and protect the heart in myocardial infarction. However, physicians believed that beta-blockers could be dangerous in patients with congestive heart failure. The reasoning went like this:

1. The heart is a pump.
2. Beta-blockers inhibit the strength and force of that pump.
3. Congestive heart failure is weakening of the pump.
4. Don't give beta-blockers to a weak pump; they will make it worse.

Logical and sound reasoning. But wrong.

In the 1980s and 1990s, scientists hypothesized that particular drugs known as calcium channel blocking medications should improve mortality in congestive heart failure or myocardial infarction. As it turned out, they did not help. However, in a subset analysis of the data, scientists found that beta-blockers lowered mortality in congestive heart failure. That did not make sense. It was axiomatic that beta-blockers were dangerous in congestive heart failure. But researchers continued to investigate, and what they found was that beta-blockers do in fact work. It turns out that beta-blockers benefit the heart simply by making it beat less frequently. Coronary arteries fill during the rest phase of the cardiac cycle. By slowing the heart rate, beta-blockers allow much more blood to fill the coronary arteries and supply the heart with tasty, nutritious oxygen. Deeelicious!

Oh, and that's not all. For the low, low price of one drug, not only do you get more oxygen supply, but we also throw in, at no extra cost to you, decreased oxygen consumption.

"Wow, Conrad, all for that one low, low price? I can't believe it."

Yes, believe it. When the heart contracts, it consumes oxygen. If you decrease the number of contractions, you decrease the demand for oxygen and, at the same time, increase the supply. It's like discovering an oil well in your backyard and switching to solar power at the same time.

"Wow, Conrad, that's amazing!"

Yes, and it doesn't stop there. As a final offer, we also throw in . . . your life! Science has shown that most patients who use beta-blockers increase survival from congestive heart failure.

"That's great, Conrad. I'll buy it! Just one question: can you refund to me all those people I knew who died because they didn't get the drug?"

WHEN I FIRST started teaching board review classes in the early 1990s, and for years after, I told students—thousands of people who are now your doctors—that beta-blockers were dangerous in congestive heart failure. How many deaths did I contribute to by mouthing the unexamined party line? Probably not more than a few hundred. My entire profession? Probably a few hundred thousand, or a million. Let's see.

Congestive heart failure is the most common admitting diagnosis in the country.

Beta-blockers have been fully approved and available since the 1960s.

They were withheld in congestive failure for decades.

We never tested beta-blockers in congestive failure, because we believed we already knew what we would find. But a funny thing happened on the way to using calcium blockers in myocardial infarction. By accident, researchers discovered something that helped congestive heart failure. They could have said, "This can't be true. We all know beta-blockers are dangerous in congestive heart failure." They could have simply discarded the evidence. But they did not. They followed up on the accident, and now we save lives with beta-blockers in congestive heart failure. This is a colossal breakthrough.

Sometimes the problem in medicine is in not following our own precepts, which are to conduct experiments, to collect data, to analyze, to find results, to repeat experiments, to confirm the results. The most damaging thing a person can do as a scientist is to speculate on results and never actually experiment to prove them. The main reason that Europeans did not cross the Atlantic until 1492 was not that they thought the Earth was flat. They just thought they knew what they would find there: India and Asia. Why go? We know what is there. It is just too far to go that way.

By going a different way, researchers showed that beta-blockers produce a whopping decrease in mortality of patients with congestive heart failure. The drug we had around for decades and withheld because we thought it was dangerous, turned out to be the most beneficial. Not only that, the weaker the heart is and the worse the function, the greater the mortality benefit. The entire reasoning that a weak heart would be harmed by beta-blockers is in fact exactly the opposite. The weaker the heart, the better the drug works? Yes, that's right! As the ejection fraction (EF)—the amount of blood pumped out with each beat—lowers, the mortality benefit increases. A normal EF is around 60 to 70 percent. When the EF drops to 40 percent, there is a 10 to 20 percent mortality benefit to the prescription of beta-blockers. When it is down to 30 percent, the benefit rises to 30 to 35 percent. When the heart is the absolute sickest, and the EF drops as low as 10 or 20 percent, the mortality benefit rises to 50 percent. Not only were we wrong, we were really, really wrong.

For 200 years, doctors used digoxin without evidence of improved mortality, solely because authority figures said to use it. It is only since the 1970s that there has been a massive uptick in the devotion to evidence-based medicine. Evidence-based medicine is such a critical advance that it is, in fact, more important than any single drug, test, or treatment in this book. The very process of how we think has shifted. We doctors no longer practice according to what some authority figure told us; instead we practice according to science, evidence, and data. How do we know something works? Because we studied it, that's why.

The quintessential tools of evidence-based medicine are statistics and the randomized controlled clinical trial. The randomized trial is only 50 years old. It has taken decades for the idea to catch on, but it is finally safe to say that all new drugs developed since the 1970s have been held to a much higher standard of evidence before approval, compared with drugs before then. Hence, ACE inhibitors were systematically studied, measured, and proven.

Thanks to evidence-based medicine, spironolactone, a diuretic, was found in 1999 to lower mortality by about 25 percent in congestive heart failure. Spironolactone is an inhibitor of aldosterone, a naturally occurring hormone produced in our adrenal glands that absorbs sodium and water and helps maintain blood pressure. Aldosterone accumulates in patients with congestive heart failure, and this is part of the reason they get fluid overload. Once it finally became clear that the problem in congestive heart failure is an overactivation of the angiotensin-aldosterone system, it was clear that spironolactone should be studied—not speculated about, but studied. Apparently we can learn from our mistakes.

JASON LAZAR AND I talk about ineffective therapies and wrong ideas. The most common cause of death immediately after a myocardial infarction is an arrhythmia, often preceded by premature ventricular contractions (PVCs).

As Jason tells it, "In the 1980s, they beat it into us with a stick: 'PVCs are bad, PVCs are bad, PVCs are bad.' A whole range of PVC suppressants was developed. We did a huge clinical trial, the Cardiac Arrhythmia Suppression Trial, or CAST. CAST was the cool, hip idea of the eighties in cardiology. 'Don't wait for arrhythmias to develop. Put everyone on an antiarrhythmic medication after a heart attack.' Oops! Guess what happened? The people who got the antiarrhythmic encainide or flecainide had triple the mortality when compared with those who received a placebo. Encainide was taken off the market, and flecainide is used now under extremely limited circumstances, and never as prophylactic therapy. What we learned is that surrogate markers are not always accurate. Surrogate markers means finding something you can measure as a predictor of who will do badly and a marker for treatment. PVCs were a surrogate marker, we thought, for people who would not do well. We successfully suppressed them. It did not help, and, in fact, made it worse."

What we learned from the CAST is that you must do a trial before anything can go into widespread use. The trial was not completed, because a group of people monitoring the data detected the problem early and stopped it. Encainide was a failure as a medication. But the evidence-based method is a resounding success. It helps physicians detect bad drugs early and discard them before they become widely available. It means that the drugs your doctor is using routinely are safe and effective. It means that there can never be another useless or toxic medication lingering on the books.

I am happy to say that evidence-based benefits in the management of congestive heart failure far outweigh evidence-based failures. There are two therapies in particular that are based on good evidence derived from systematic study. One is the implantation of the cardioverter defibrillator in patients with weak heart muscles from insufficient blood flow. The most common cause of death after a myocardial infarction is an arrhythmia, and it is sudden. If you have a low ejection fraction, we do not wait around for you to have your first potentially fatal arrhythmia after an infarction. We put in the implantable defibrillator.

The other breakthrough is the implantation of biventricular pacemakers in patients with dilated cardiomyopathy and a delay in conduction in the cardiac conduction system. If your electrocardiogram (EKG) shows a wide QRS complex (the measurement of the Q, R, and S waves), we put in a biventricular pacemaker and resynchronize the heart.

Jason tells me about another of the "unsexy" advances in his area. High blood pressure, or hypertension, is the most common disease in the United States. For the last half century or more, physicians and other health care providers have almost exclusively monitored blood pressure. Now, it turns out that physicians scare people: blood pressure measured by a physician is higher than it would be normally. Home blood pressure monitoring can show a blood pressure 10 full points lower than what would be found if measured in the doctor's office. It turns out many doctors are using blood pressure medications to treat a physical manifestation of anxiety. Home blood pressure monitoring is a huge advance that has been thought about for years, yet the American College of Cardiology did not officially endorse it until 2008.

DR. JEFFREY BORER is director of cardiology at SUNY Downstate. He is at the absolute top of the food chain when it comes to cardiology. Besides being a fully functional clinical cardiologist, he is arguably the world's leading authority on valvular heart disease. In addition, as the chairman of the advisory committee on new cardiac devices for the Food and Drug Administration, he is as well informed as any man alive. He is also an elegant, warm man who smiles readily and puts me instantly at ease. He reminds me of my grandmother's general practitioner, who, when I was a child, would visit the house and have a cup of tea. He has the old-school charm of a doctor making a house call and the cutting-edge intelligence of a scientist on the verge of the next breakthrough.

In the future, the cardiologist will carry a black bag that is like a doorway into another dimension. That dimension is the infinite cosmos of the human genome, or DNA, and the mysteries contained within it. Into that bag will go a sample of the patient's genetic structure, and out of it will come individualized medicine.

"The future of cardiology," says Dr. Jeffrey Borer, "lies in the application of molecular methods to real, live human beings. The future will see us analyzing the individual genetic characteristics of each patient and planning treatments around what we know will happen to that person as time goes on. I know you are a 'drama' guy, Conrad, and the concept of prevention may not have the kind of drama you are looking for to make people feel grateful for what they have, but it is the truth nevertheless. It's great to be able to give people a thrombolytic to bust open a clot, but it is greater to make sure they never have the clot to begin with."

Jeff exudes such magnetic personal warmth that it is a while before I realize he has both disagreed with me and criticized me. But his charm forces me to admire him for the beauty with which I have just found out my focus is wrong.

In the future that Jeff Borer is sculpting for this country, a man like my heart-diseased friend Father John Collins, whose story I told in the preface to this book, will have his genetic structure analyzed. Specific therapies and lifestyle modifications will be suggested for him years before he has a twinge of pain in the swimming pool. Prevention is a hard sell to legislators, insurers, and the public. A quarter-million dollars for an organ transplant inspires drama. It compels us. A priest about to pass out and drown in a pool inspires a passionate, immediate intervention. A few dollars and a few office visits years before my friend's coronary stenosis developed are not as compelling.

We tend to fund the things that compel us. We have a clear track record of legislation in service of illness. Diseases like kidney failure and AIDS have captivated the political will of the country, and by legislative effort—boom!—we had universal coverage. We have the money if we decide to make it a priority.

Jeff discusses the case of my friend Father Collins: "With his family history, the future molecular specialist would see this myocardial infarction coming a million miles off and take steps to intervene. Our job is to get the people who fund health care—the legislators and insurers—to understand that a few dollars spent on medication, exercise, and diet are worth way more than the thousands spent on procedures." If a physician spends five hours educating the patient on how to prevent heart disease, this is barely valued. If the physician spends five hours doing surgery to reverse disease that is already life-threatening, the reimbursement is hugely greater.

In between the genes that we know code for identifiable human elements, such as blue eyes or the number of fingers we have, is a vast ocean of unknown genetic data and sequences. When you ask geneticists what the stuff in between is for, they say "nothing" or "old viruses that got sucked into our chromosomes" or "Extra stuff with no purpose." Imagine visiting Manhattan landmarks like the Statue of Liberty and the Empire State Building and the Metropolitan Museum of Art and then asking your tour guide what the other spaces in between are for. If the guide were to say "nothing" or "extra stuff with no purpose," what would you think? In Manhattan, real estate is at a premium; no matter how compact it is, it is prime real estate that must contain something. The human genome is like prime real estate. It is, in fact, precisely the amount of unknown information that characterizes the higher life forms — that is, you and me. What possibilities lie within?

A bacterium contains a lot of coding sequences. Every single piece of DNA in a bacterium is known to code for something identifiable. There is no "extra." What you see is what you get. No unknown. No extra. No possibilities. The difference between a mouse, a fruit fly, an *E coli* bacterium, and us is not so much the number of known elements but rather the amount of the unknown. What cure is hidden there? Are the sequences for the next saint, poet, opera singer there? Or the sequences for telepathy and visions? The fundamental nature of the human being, genetically speaking, lies in having the greatest amount of unknown possibilities.

In terms of cardiology, Jeff Borer says, "The greatest paradigm shift will be the use of molecular, genetic medicine."

This book is largely about the drama of amazing new procedures that reverse disease. Procedures and treatments that, prior to even ten years ago, you would have had to be a biblical figure to perform. It also aims to sell the idea of prevention, to make it sexy enough to get it funded and reimbursed.

CONGESTIVE HEART FAILURE and hypertension are among the most prevalent illnesses in the United States. The last ten years have seen the most extraordinary triumphs in this area. From 1782 to 1981 we had one drug with no mortality benefit, digoxin, plus diuretics to relieve symptoms; from 1981 to 1997 we had one drug that had a proven mortality benefit; then there was a sudden rocket launch in 1998, leading us to the present: three classes of drugs that lower mortality (ACE inhibitors, beta-blockers, and spironolactone) and two devices that lower mortality (the implantable defibrillator and the biventricular pacemaker). In other words, more has come out in the last 10 years to save lives and improve symptoms from congestive heart failure than in the history of mankind. And yet the majority of medical students think that it was better to be in medicine 25 years ago, when we did not have any drugs to lower mortality in the most common admitting diagnosis in the country, when we were actually withholding a lifesaving medication, and when we routinely used a toxic medication.

Dr. Jason Lazar outlines some of the most critical advances in the history of medicine, making Hippocrates look like a third-rate hack. Yet he doesn't express any sense of happiness or excitement or hope about them. In fact, he is reticent and almost embarrassed not to have anything "sexy" to offer. His patients hardly notice the advances. Preventive medicine is not dramatic. You do not notice it when you fail to die. Jason has become inured to miracles because they are routine. But we are at this moment offering the best therapy in the history of the world in service of a suffering humanity.

And that, Jason, is a sexy thing indeed.

From year to year my hopes of being cured have gradually been shattered . . . I must live like an outcast; if I appear in company, I am overcome by a burning anxiety, a fear that I am running the risk of letting people notice my condition . . . How humiliated I have felt if somebody standing beside me heard the sound of a flute in the distance and I heard nothing.

—Ludwig van Beethoven

CHAPTER 11

Reversing Deafness

"In an Hour, Fifteen Years of Misery Were Stopped"

YOU POSSESS ONE of the most extraordinary pieces of engineering in the known universe. When a sound wave hits your ear, it causes the eardrum, or tympanic membrane, to vibrate. A series of three minute bones known as ossicles transmits these vibrations to the inner ear. The ossicles include the stapes, which, at about three millimeters long, is the smallest bone in the human body. Movement of the stapes creates a wave of gentle, fluid motion that goes into the inner ear, or cochlea. The cochlea looks like a seashell, becoming progressively narrower as it turns. Minute hair cells inside the cochlea bend like seaweed swaying gently in the current on the ocean floor. When they bend, they send an electrical signal to the auditory nerve, which transmits these electrical signals into the brain stem, where the nucleus of the auditory nerve will convert them into chemicals. These chemical neurotransmitters go into the brain to be perceived as sound.

When I was a medical student, I thought I was going to be an ear specialist. Until I beheld the mysterious grandeur of the inner ear, I had classified myself as an agnostic. Now I had to wonder. The existence of the inner ear was, to me, the best circumstantial evidence I had so far for the existence of a Creator.

BEFORE MEETING OLGA LIS, director of audiology at Long Island College Hospital in Brooklyn, I had already interviewed five attending specialists in otolaryngology (the study of the ear, nose, and throat). They ranged from fellowship-trained ear surgeons to the chair of a department. They were all faculty at a large medical school. I initially found it strange that they were deferring most of my questions to an audiologist: "You will have to ask Olga," "Olga knows the best," "We just put in the cochlear implant, Olga does all the training," "Olga knows." This was the constant refrain. Why, I wondered, are all the team captains and generals deferring to some glorified technician?

When I meet Olga, I understand in a flash. If the surgeon is the commander in chief and the department chair the general, then this audiologist is a member of the Special Forces. I am sitting in the audiology testing room, the door or which closes with a definitive effect. Olga sizes me up in about three milliseconds.

"Here is a book on implants," she says. "Here are three DVDs of explanations, and here is a list of patients with their exact procedure listed. Hold out your hand. This is one of the devices. I have told each person you will be calling. Any questions?"

Olga is perfectly manicured. Her speech is precise. Now I know why the specialists all defer to her.

Olga Lis programs cochlear implants, electronic devices that are inserted directly into the ear in order to convert a deaf person into someone who can hear. The surgical placement of a cochlear implant is the simplest part. The doctor basically makes a little cut in the skin, drills a little hole into the auditory nerve, and attaches a wire. If the auditory nerve is missing, the surgeon can put the receiver directly into the brain stem. That in itself is miraculous. But the real work is in mapping and programming the device. *Mapping* means determining the precise threshold at which sounds are perceived. Mapping also allows the patient to learn what the sounds actually mean. Otherwise, what the patient perceives is just noise. Olga is the one who first diagnoses hearing loss and later teaches the recipient of a cochlear implant how to recognize speech.

You may think it a simple matter to diagnose hearing loss, but it can be very difficult, especially in a small child. You can put an adult patient in a soundproof chamber, like an underwater bathysphere, and ask if he or she can hear a series of progressively louder beeps. You cannot, however, conduct such a test with a child under the age of three. Small children cannot just say, "Mother, dear, I do believe my high-frequency hearing perception is impaired." And early diagnosis of hearing loss in a child is critical, because if a child does not hear language by the age of five or six, he or she may never learn to speak.

The ability to speak is largely based on the ability of a child to hear. Olga says, "When Abigail was brought to me, it was for a 'third opinion.' Her parents were originally told her hearing was normal. Another audiologist felt different. When I met her, it was totally clear: this child was deaf."

Abigail has a genetic defect known as Mondini's deformity, which is an abnormal shortening of the cochlea. In such cases, the cochlea is like an instrument missing its essential parts, a clarinet without holes, a guitar without strings, a French horn without its turns. Mondini's deformity is a progressive cause of deafness.

Olga says that by the time Abigail's parents, Sandra and Trevor Dyer, came to her, it was clear immediately that their child needed an implant. If Abigail did not get an implant soon, her speech might be forever abnormal.

"Her mother was nine months pregnant at the time," Olga says, "and she was on board with it. Her father was not. Trevor is a very religious person . . . They were looking for divine intervention."

"I thought that God would take care of her," Trevor later says to me. "He created her this way, and He could fix what was wrong with her . . . I thought God would heal her supernaturally. Here she is, my beautiful little girl, and I was afraid of the stigma of the hearing aids, and I was afraid of the stigma of the implant. We prayed and went to church, and people prayed over her. I thought it would be like in the Bible where the woman with the issue of blood touches Jesus on the hem of his garment and she is healed . . . I thought Jesus would touch her on the ear and she would be healed without human intervention."

Trevor continues, "I went to see Dr. Sperling, and I talked this over with him."

Dr. Neil Sperling is the otolaryngologist at the center of the work on restoring hearing, a specialist in ear surgery at Long Island College Hospital in New York City. If you want a physician of intensely high skill who can operate through a keyhole slit a few millimeters across and replace the minute ossicles of the ear with titanium parts, then you go see Dr. Sperling. His patients call Dr. Sperling a miracle worker. I interview a dozen of them, and far more than one, even the calmest among them, say the same thing in the same words.

I pass the summary of my dozen patient interviews on to Dr. Sperling. I am disappointed. It is almost as if he thinks I am talking about someone else.

"The most gratifying thing to me is to see patients in the office after a procedure and to see that their hearing is much better," he says.

Either he is refractory to the "miracle worker" label or it makes him uncomfortable. Or perhaps he is just one of those sober-minded medical practitioners who eschews euphoric verbiage.

He says, "I suppose if in someone's belief system they think of it as a miracle, that is good for them. Cochlear implant surgery, although it may result in a dramatic improvement in hearing for the patient, is certainly not a complex procedure. Placing the implant is not technically demanding. It is rather straightforward."

I don't think Dr. Sperling sees the disappointed look on my face. "Are you aware, Dr. Sperling, that Trevor Dyer changed his mind to do the implant on his daughter because of what you said in this regard? Mr. Dyer says you told him, 'This is the miracle you have been waiting for.'"

"I said that?"

"Yes," I reply. "And that phrase is what he remembers as having changed his mind."

DEAF CHILDREN AND their families have to spend a lot of time with Olga Lis. They have to visit her office many times to progressively increase the amount of stimulus and sound the patient perceives so that he or she can make sense of it. For a two-year-old who has always been deaf, hearing can be quite frightening at first. When you receive an implant, you don't just switch it on and start appreciating Beethoven. There is a lot of work that must be completed before such a thing can happen.

"After a long time, the children eventually come to hear even nuances in voice. Over time, they hear and understand more and more. One day, they hear enough and they suddenly say to me, 'Oh! You have an accent!' When they say this, my job is done." Olga is a Russian immigrant. She has perfect English and only a trace remnant of an accent.

"You know, it's funny how things turn out," Trevor says. "The other day Abigail heard me and her brother talking about another child who is deaf. Abigail is eight now."

"She came over and asked, 'What does *deaf* mean, Daddy?'"

Hearing Trevor now, I find it hard to believe that he nearly rejected Abigail's implant. He is ebullient about all the new technology. He bubbles over with details about devices, methods, and the organizational plans of deaf schools.

"Do you know that the teachers are in class with a microphone around their neck that goes straight into the implants of the children?" he asks, almost levitating out of his chair. "No matter how far they are away, the children can hear the teacher because there is a wireless system that goes right to their ears."

Trevor would agree that we are living in the age of miracles. They pour out of our hands. In addition to being religious, Trevor and Sandra Dyer are talkative people, and we have a long theological discussion.

"So," I ask Trevor at one point, "were your prayers for Abigail answered, just not in the form you expected? Was it in the form of electrical impulses reaching the ear with a frequency of 120,000 per second? Did Jesus touch her on the ear?"

Trevor says, "That is exactly it."

Sandra chimes in, "Knock, and the door shall be opened."

PERHAPS GOD IS here all the time. My own belief is that divine and cosmic forces of goodness do reach the Earth, but it is up to humanity to receive and transmit them. I rarely stop for anything, and I barely listen, yet I have only to tilt my head and leap up to catch a forward pass from the Divine Guy. The implementation of miracles is up to us. But for many physicians the desire to implement is hindered by paperwork, preapprovals, denials of reimbursement for legitimate care, and the disgusting feeling of haggling over money with the insurance system.

Dr. Sperling points out, "I really think there is a force of mediocritization of medicine. There is every reason [in this insurance system] not to do things that require extra effort. There is every reason for me to do less and not to do more. There is no reward from insurers to go the extra mile. There is no value placed on that from the system. There is no reward for taking care of very complicated patients. There are specialists who are taking care of simple cases and just removing the wax from patients' ears all day long, and they are doing very well. They are doing a very basic practice. That is absolutely rewarded in our system.

There is no value placed on exceptional work and involving yourself in complicated patients. They take more time, and the insurance system at present actually seems to punish you for it."

Dr. Sperling's patients may describe his work in restoring and improving their hearing as miraculous, yet he feels like the system is punishing him for taking on tough cases. He sees a system of insurers that rewards mediocrity, not excellence. He is not looking for more money or nice letters of appreciation. His patients are already highly appreciative. All he wants is to improve the system of health care delivery so that he does not have to fight the insurance companies and the patients' diseases at the same time. One day Dr. Sperling may well decide to retire early because it is just too much of a hassle to practice medicine. Who will suffer?

We will. Rescuing the physician from the bureaucracy of managed care is the same as rescuing our own future health.

I want to make the blessings of our technology so apparent that even the most fiscally conservative will long to expand insurance coverage of them to include everyone in our society. Dr. Sperling and his colleagues need expanded health insurance coverage and more funding for research in hearing disorders. Even a person immune to a sense of miracles can see that, with a 60 percent unemployment rate among the deaf, the cost of the implant is minuscule compared to lost earnings. The cost of an implant—including the device itself, the follow-up visits, the mapping, and the training—is between $35,000 and $60,000. Compare that to a lifetime spent out of the workforce, not contributing to the tax base but instead drawing Social Security insurance or disability payments. Lifetime earnings for a hearing-impaired person are between $300,000 and $600,000 less than those of a person with normal hearing.

In addition to economic benefits, the development of an improved and more readily available cochlear implant would be a boost to the military. The tympanic membrane is highly susceptible to the wave of air pressure a bomb produces. The most common nonlethal injury from a roadside bomb or an improvised explosive device is hearing impairment.

Deaf soldiers cannot function. They are discharged. The cost of their training is wasted, and they are maintained on disability payments for the rest of their lives. Doubling the funding for the National Institute on Deafness and Other Communication Disorders every five years is in the interest of national security. Is it a far leap to say that your elected official is a participant in the performance of miraculous events?

HERE'S ANOTHER PUZZLER: What kills more people in the United States each year, shark attacks or coconuts? You are probably guessing that it must be coconuts or I would not be asking. Falling coconuts result in far more injury and death than shark attacks. You are lying on the beach enjoying your piña colada when—*bang!*—a falling coconut nails you. The coconut causes head trauma and intracranial bleeding. Perhaps if Steven Spielberg were to make a big-budget movie called *Coconuts,* there would be greater public awareness of this fact.

Public health researchers study what it is that is actually killing and injuring us. Unfortunately, time, money, and national resources are sometimes devoted instead to things that are not causing such harm. Otosclerosis, a disease resulting in deafness, is a major underfunded cause of suffering and disability for more than a million Americans. Otosclerosis is an overgrowth of the bones of the middle ear, so that the normally moving stapes becomes entrapped. This hardening damages the system that conducts sound through the middle ear. It takes years to progress. Slowly, slowly, your ear is strangled off from sound. It is very likely what made Beethoven deaf.

When I talk to Jose Santos about the 15 years he lost to deafness, I am especially touched by his lack of anger or resentment. Only when I press him does Jose express his negative feelings.

"I did not go out, I couldn't participate in conversations, I did not want to do anything," he says. "I hated having to ask everyone to repeat themselves, so I just stayed alone. Life went on around me, and I was an observer—a depressed observer. For fifteen years I tried every type of hearing aid, but all it did was make louder sounds that I could not really understand. The hardest thing for me is that I could not hear my grandson cooing."

Through a minute laser incision around the tympanic membrane, our miracle worker, Dr. Neil Sperling, takes less than an hour to remove the bone that has for 15 years been engulfing Jose Santos's stapes. Without even an overnight stay in the hospital, Jose walks out the door and hears the world.

Surgical stapedectomy has been around for a long time, but the ability to use a laser, to do the surgery smaller, with less recovery time and faster results, is new. When I first spoke to Dr. Sperling, he did not expect Mr. Santos to be a good candidate for me to talk to. The procedure had been done nearly five years before. He expected Jose Santos to have forgotten the pain of his deafness and the miracle of a laser stapedectomy.

But to this day, Mr. Santos says, "Dr. Sperling is a miracle worker. Everything is different, everything . . . In an hour, fifteen years of misery were stopped. I came off the table, and my life was restored back to me. It was instantaneous. I went into the hospital cut off and separate. Miserable and depressed. I left the hospital on the same day happy. I felt like I rejoined the world, but I guess it is better to say that the world rejoined me."

He never brings up the fact that his diagnosis was missed, although he does says that during his 15 years of deafness he begged his doctors to do something. He never, even when pressed, expresses anger at those who did not do the procedure earlier. I have listened to his interview tapes a dozen times, and I am still pondering his complete lack of resentment. I get the feeling that he is now always at the opera. Jose is, apparently, too busy enjoying music, movies, and the voices of his grandchildren to dwell on negative emotions.

Jose tells me, "Last year I gave away my hearing aids."

In the interviews I conduct for this book, "almost miraculous" is the mildest phrase people use to describe laser stapedectomy. The technique produces such instant results that sounds come flooding in. I do not prompt people to talk about miracles. I do not ask leading questions such as "Is this miraculous?" They volunteer the language of miracles even though all I ask is for them to talk about their treatment.

I want all the Jose Santoses of the world to hear their grandchildren, and all the mothers to hear their children.

"I FELT LIKE I had bionic ears," says Tina McKinnley-Page.

It took two years for Tina to get diagnosed correctly. She was only in her late twenties when she became impaired with the hearing loss you would expect in an older person. Otosclerosis is twice as common in women as in men. We don't know why.

"I did not know it was happening at first," Tina says. "Then it got a lot worse during my pregnancy."

Otosclerosis can get much worse during pregnancy. We don't know why. My guess is that society has not determined that deaf pregnant women are enough of a priority to fully study it.

WE DON'T KNOW what causes otosclerosis, but we do know that it can be inherited. If you have one parent with otosclerosis, you have a 25 percent chance of having otosclerosis. If you have two parents with it, then you have a 50 percent chance of having otosclerosis.

Suzanne White is a New York City schoolteacher. Her mother and sister have otosclerosis. One grandfather had it. So it is no surprise that Ms. White herself underwent a laser stapedectomy.

She says, "After the procedure, it all comes to you in intense clarity. It is almost scary. I could hear my cell phone ringing on another floor. I could hear what was being said from another person's cell phone. But the most important thing for me is that I can hear if someone is in need."

In the hundreds of interviews I have conducted, I have not found a single person exaggerating an illness or disability for a secondary gain. I have found no one feigning helplessness so that a difficulty in functioning will be excused. I have found, however, many individuals trying to hide their disabilities. I have found examples of shame. Patients want to feel they can measure up and function at the same level or a better level than their peers at work and in the family. No one wants to be lesser than others. No one wants to feel he or she is a burden on others. The worst fear for some is not being able to hear well enough to protect family members in the event of an emergency.

AN EDUCATOR LIKE Suzanne White, Nate Kohlmann was also most concerned about his ability to take care of other people.

A 30-year-old assistant principal in a New York City school, he says, "I had a series of ear problems my entire life. I had procedures done that didn't work. I was losing my hearing. Do you know how embarrassing it is for children who are already shy to have to be told to repeat themselves three times in a classroom?"

Repeated childhood infections destroyed the bones of Nate's middle ear. He had drainage tubes put in, and the holes did not heal over.

"I had to plug my ears when I took a shower," he says. "I couldn't get water in them. I couldn't go swimming. I had to make sure people always sat on the right side of me, or I couldn't hear them. It was frustrating. I was always misunderstanding people."

Even the nonchalant Dr. Neil Sperling expresses some amazement at the procedure he is able to perform for Nate: "Reconstructing the middle ear requires real skill that is rare and hard to achieve. We use titanium implants to reconstruct the chain of ossicles. You have to work in an amazingly small space. This is a high level of craftsmanship."

Imagine operating down a canal less than an inch in diameter and manipulating bones that are so small that a half millimeter either way is the difference between deafness and hearing. Like a watchmaker, Dr. Sperling has put in place and lined up tiny pieces of titanium, constructed like the body's own ossicles, to bridge the gap between Nate's eardrum and the receptive apparatus underneath, the cochlea.

Nate reports, "My hearing increased exponentially. I was able to function. I could hear the children."

If the ossicles are frozen, we have laser stapedectomy to free them. If the ossicles can't be freed or if they have been destroyed, as were Nate's, we have ossicular chain reconstruction, so that sound impulses can travel to the cochlea of the inner ear and then to the auditory nerve. If the cochlea is damaged, we have cochlear implants to attach a receiver and wire to the cochlea and the auditory nerve. If the auditory nerve is destroyed—if there is simply nothing to receive impulses on that side of the head—we have a titanium implant surgically placed in the bone on the side of the hearing loss from the destroyed nerve. Bone grows around the implant and permanently fixes the implant in the skull. A transceiver is placed next to the ear. Sound is perceived and relayed to the titanium implant, or bone-anchored hearing aid (BAHA). The sound is then conducted through the skull, through the bone to the opposite side of the head, and the auditory nerve on the other side of the head picks up the sound. It is essentially like adding an ear back on one side of the head where there was none.

IN ORDER TO LOCATE where sounds are coming from, two ears are necessary. When you have two ears, you can localize the sound. With only one, if someone shouts at you, you will not know which direction to turn. Also, having two ears helps diminish background noise.

After a car accident that ripped off part of her head, Anita was left with one ear. She was in a coma for three weeks.

"I was expected to die," she says. "Please don't use my last name. People I work with don't know I had this much damage to my ear. I work in the resource room at school, and I don't want people to know that I couldn't function."

Hers is one of the few requests for anonymity I received in the course of doing interviews for this book.

"I don't want pity," she adds, and then continues: "I felt very blessed not to have died and not to have my brain damaged. I felt lucky. But then I started to realize how hard it was to function without hearing on that side. It was hard to rush down to meetings in the principal's office to make sure I got there first so I would get the right seat so I could hear things correctly. It was embarrassing to always ask people to repeat things, and I did not want people to know. I did not want people to think of me as disabled."

As I listen, I wonder how many people I come across in my daily life who are hiding a disability that they are ashamed of.

Doctors replaced Anita's ossicles with titanium implants mixed with bone. Anita now says, "I hear perfectly well in both ears." Spontaneously she adds, "I thank God for blessing the doctors for being able to work this miracle."

"How do you know your hearing is normal, Anita?"

"Because now sometimes I hear things I don't want to hear."

MAIDIE ERICKSON'S STORY is to me like a science-fiction novel, a fairy tale, or perhaps the New Testament story of Jesus healing a deaf man (Mark 7:32–37). Who would figure that a miracle could happen on an ordinary weekday in Brooklyn?

Maidie is a highly intelligent engineer who is often the only woman on a construction site with loud, heavy equipment. She is a "Sand Hog" digging a water tunnel under the island of Manhattan.

"I could not locate sounds," she says. "Without two ears I could not hear where things were coming from. It was kind of a pain in the ass, really, but I never thought of myself as disabled. My mother said God made me special. She never allowed me to think of myself as disabled. Wherever I went, I had to have people sit on my left side so I could hear."

When Maidie was born, her right ear looked a little small but not extraordinarily so. Only when you took a closer look could you see the problem: there was no ear canal, no way for sound to travel inside to the nerves to be perceived by her brain.

Now there is.

Dr. Neil Sperling approaches this achievement with the same matter-of-fact manner that he does his other work. I sit in the presence of a man who carved an ear canal into the side of a young woman's head and made her a new ear.

He says very plainly, "We constructed a new tympanic membrane and took skin from her buttock and made the skin of the canal."

Maidie already had a functioning auditory nerve buried in her head. She had the minute series of three ossicles, but they were not connected to anything from the outside.

"Dr. Sperling says the audiogram showed that I had hearing in there, but I could never hear anything through it," she says. "When I got an infection in my normal ear, I could not hear anything. I had heard of the possibility of reconstructing the ear, but it was always too risky or expensive to try it. When Dr. Sperling told me about the procedure, he warned me that there was no guarantee. It might work or it might not.

"When I came off the table, I could hear everything. It is like living your whole life thinking there was only one dimension, then you find out all of a sudden there are three dimensions that everyone knew about but you did not. In an instant, my entire concept of normal changed. For me, I had never heard the real world before, but that was 'normal' for me. Now I knew what everyone else was hearing. My family was overwhelmed."

Maidie describes the event from what I imagine to be the point of view of a child being born, from the point of view of finding out about the existence of a world you never knew was there: "It was like hearing for the first time . . . It was overwhelming because everything comes into you. I know it sounds silly, but I did not know my refrigerator clicks on and off. I did not know how to shut the world off. It was like having hearing ADD [attention deficit disorder] . . . A normal person's brain learns how to filter all of this out."

At this point in my research, I have done 175 patient interviews. For me, each interview is a little like reading about the mystical experience of someone who, through meditation and effort, breaks through into some radical new understanding. In the last 20 or 30 years, we as a society have accumulated colossal benefits in medicine. We have so much goodness to bestow on a suffering humanity that I am overwhelmed with the impulse to extend these benefits universally to the entire population. Until that happens, contemplation of the availability of goodness I am describing can be a solvent for the insensitivity of jaded caregivers.

"I could hear people talking half a football field away," Maidie says. "On the job, they call me Wonder Woman because I have bionic hearing." She adds, "I did not know that you could hear bass and treble at the same time. I did not know that normal people could hear their own breathing. I know it sounds small, but having a stereo became the coolest thing ever."

Many people I interview, including Maidie, start out saying they do not know how to describe their experience or they don't have much to say. In not a single interview so far has a patient been the one to stop talking. In every case, it is up to me to draw the conversation to a close.

Maidie, like so many others, has an endless ability to find words for her happiness. What she says is like poetry: "I could hear every bird chirping. I could hear the crinkling of my clothes, every whisper, I could hear everything, and it was overwhelming."

CHAPTER 12

Nurture the Next Generation

Ophthalmology Depends on Obsolescence

D R. DOUGLAS LAZZARO, the chairman of ophthalmology at SUNY Downstate, is an ebullient, boisterous man. He is the kind of guy you might see at a ball game with his face painted in his team's colors, the kind of guy who leaps up to do a cheer or throws his arms into the air to do the wave. Once he hears I am doing a book on medical advances, he stops what he is doing and grabs his cell phone to identify cool new stuff for me. It appears that his enthusiasm is causing him to talk fast, though really he's just speaking with average velocity for a New Yorker.

At 46, Doug is at the top of his game—old enough to have 20 years' experience and young enough to be learning new methods. He is a specialist in operating on the cornea. A master of his field, he runs one of the biggest residency programs in the country. And yet he's so down-to-earth you might mistake him for a first-generation college graduate. That's not the case, though: his father is a long-term faculty member in the same department. At 68, Dr. Clifford Lazzaro is an ophthalmologist whose years of experience are double those of his son.

I watch them toss a ball of excitement as they run down the different subjects in ophthalmology. I feel like the team mascot at practice with the professional ballplayers. They describe the new methods at the speed of thought.

Clifford takes the first toss, opening with the revolution in glaucoma treatment: "When I got started, all we had was two drugs, pilocarpine and epinephrine . . . The surgery that we did for glaucoma needed a fistula, or hole, made in the eye to allow drainage of the fluid out of the eye . . . The hole was cut into the iris and made a tract to the outside. This was done when the drops didn't work.

"Once I had a friend of mine I was very close to who had the procedure done. He was operated on by the best surgeon in the eastern United States. Then one day he went swimming and caught pinkeye, or conjunctivitis. For you and me, conjunctivitis means nothing, but for this person . . . the infection spread into the eye. That 'minor' infection results in him losing his eye.

"Now we use a laser to create a drainage pathway inside the eye. The laser is shot through the cornea, and the focal point is set so there is zero damage to the cornea. The focal point is the place where the energy of the laser comes to a point. It is the place of maximum transmission of energy, like the tip of a cone. The laser disperses the tissue like lightning and thunder.

"Now we have a dozen drugs. People get their glaucoma detected before it has caused any damage at all to the eye. They go on medications that prevent the need for surgery. The pharmacology of glaucoma management is completely revolutionary.

"When I was a resident, you had to stay in the hospital for a week for cataract removal. We used to open up half the eye. In 1971, when I started, you had sutures in place for weeks. It took eight weeks before we gave you these ridiculous glasses with a thickness that looked like the bottom of a bottle of Coca-Cola. Now you get a two-millimeter incision, the cataract gets removed in five minutes, and the patient goes home the same day. They cut open the cornea and pop in a foldable lens, which unfolds in place in a few seconds. Within a few days, you are completely rehabilitated and back at work. "

But wait. There's more. Clifford goes on: "Macular degeneration is the most common cause of blindness in adults. I was never impressed by the old treatments. Now, all of a sudden, you have injectable medications that completely stop it in ninety-seven percent of people. Thirty percent of people have their vision loss reversed.

"I think it is mind-blowing."

FATHER AND SON are both excited about a protocol they are writing for the prevention of migraine headaches.

I ask a dumb question: "Why are you eye doctors paying attention to migraine headaches? What's the connection?"

"Because so many of them get visual disturbances."

Doug doesn't even pause to allow me to notice that I should have thought about this. He knows that doctors are not God.

"Let me call a patient of ours to talk to you about it," suggests Doug.

During the phone conversation that follows, the patient, Douglas Carletta, tells me an amazing story.

"I used to get migraines every few months only a couple of times a year," Mr. Carletta says. "Then they started happening all the time. I got an echocardiogram, and they told me about this hole in my heart, the patent foramen ovale. I tried this new procedure. They seemed kind of hesitant at first. That was when I realized they had never done the procedure themselves before—they had only assisted at them. They put a catheter in my groin, and they put a thing in my heart that looks like a clamshell. The migraines stopped overnight. I realized I was lucky to have had this done at Miami Children's Hospital. Where the hole was, was difficult for anyone to do because it was so small, so it was good to do in a place where they were used to operating on children."

Clifford and Doug Lazzaro are publishing that case, along with another, and are working on designing a protocol to study the phenomenon. It turns out that as many as two-thirds of patients with migraines have a patent foramen ovale (PFO), the abnormal opening in the heart that I described in chapter 10. For someone with a PFO, a clot from the legs that would normally get caught in the lungs may go up to the brain.

"It is possible to close the defect with a catheter. I hope our department will be the first to describe it," says Clifford.

Here is a man who is 68 years old, an age at which other doctors might be thinking exclusively about retirement, trying to run fast enough to publish a new breakthrough first.

"I have two grandsons who have atrial septal defects and several other family members with the same defect," he says, "so the gene must be on my side. I have a cousin who is getting severe migraine headaches every two weeks. Then one day, I get called and told he is having stroke, in his thirties. They find he has the PFO, and they close it with a catheter. His migraines go away . . .

"Migraineurs are . . . crippled by their pain. This is amazingly big. A lot of people are losing a lot of work because of their pain. This procedure lessens the intensity of the pain. Can you imagine how much work is being lost by their pain, and how many billions of dollars in lost work can be fixed?"

Although I have never had a migraine, I have seen many strong, capable people laid low with them. Even though the PFO procedure is still only a possibility, you would think that doctors would be shouting it from the rooftops.

Clifford adds, "People may refuse, because of the risk as well as the time it takes to do it."

"Come on, it is a percutaneous procedure," I say. "You can get it done in the amount of time it takes to get a double soy latte at Starbucks."

Clifford Lazzaro has enough sportsmanship to laugh at my jokes.

As for Doug Carletta, the only one of us to have gone through with the procedure: "The only funny thing was I had to stay in the children's hospital overnight. When I woke up, there were clowns in the room. I was glad my migraines were gone, but I told them I did not want to do any coloring that morning."

"I NEEDED GLASSES to find my glasses," Daria Emmett tells me. "I could not see any of the eye chart without glasses. My eyesight was terrible. I was going from bifocals to trifocals. I could not see people's faces even if they were in front of me. I knew there were two eyes and a nose, but I could not recognize people. I was using glasses for thirty years. I went for the procedure at four o'clock P.M. and told my husband to pick me up at Dr. Lazzaro's office at four-thirty. By the time my husband came, I was already outside waiting for him. "

Daria at this point is nearly bouncing off the chair with the excitement building in her voice. I am not used to this. I am usually the one reminding people of the specialness of their procedures.

"At the end of the procedure they'd told me to keep my eyes closed, but I couldn't help myself," she says. "I . . . started cheating by opening my eyes. Within ten minutes of the procedure, I was reading the license plates off the cars in front of us without glasses. How cool is that?" But then she adds, "After the procedure, I was scared."

"Of what?" I ask, fearing some disaster.

"When something is so good and you don't want it to end, you are scared it will go away."

She is so ecstatic that I wonder for a moment if this is a patient with a delusional disorder. Is this how I come across to other people when I start getting excited about advances in medicine?

Daria starts to laugh out of the blue.

"What's so funny?" I ask.

"Well, it's just that I still keeping reaching up to push on my glasses. I don't wear glasses anymore, but I am still pushing up on them even though they are not there."

Daria is the beneficiary of a laser in-situ keratomileusis (LASIK) operation. LASIK corrects a refractive error, which is the collective term for both nearsightedness (myopia) and farsightedness (hyperopia).

Doug Lazzaro goes into detail about LASIK: "The cornea is only about half a millimeter, or 500 microns, thick at the center of the eye in front. We use an excimer laser to slice off a flap of the cornea. The layer is only about 120 microns thick. It's an important 120 microns, though—it contains all the pain receptors and nerve endings. This flap is the reason the procedure is not painful. After the flap is lifted up, we use a femtosecond laser to do the work to reshape the cornea."

"What's a femto second laser?" I ask, thinking that there must have been a femto first laser and somehow I'd missed it.

"No, Conrad, it's *femtosecond*. It's a laser that pulses at one-quadrillionth of a second."

Damn, that sounds small. It is. Another way of writing it is 0.00000000000001 second.

"LASIK has been approved for about fifteen years," says Doug, "but now we have the ability to track the iris so that if the eye has oscillations, or movements, the laser will follow it. It uses the same technology that the military uses to precisely guide missiles. It keeps the laser focused by using infrared tracking. It is revolutionary."

By keeping the laser focused on the iris, the surgeon can lock in the pupil. If the surgeon locks in the laser on the right spot, so that there are no oscillations, then the accuracy is extraordinary.

"After we reshape the cornea, we put the flap back down to cover the front of the eye," Doug says. "Since the flap has the nerve endings, and we don't damage it, that is why the procedure won't hurt." If you touch the surface of the eye, it hurts; if you lift up the flap of the front of the eye with all the nerve endings, it will not hurt.

The U.S. Food and Drug Administration (FDA) approved LASIK because of its remarkable clinical study results. One year after the procedure, 100 percent of the clinical study participants could pass a driving test without glasses or contacts; 98 percent could see 20/20 or better without glasses or contacts; and 70 percent could see 20/16 or better without glasses or contacts. Moreover, compared to the control group (the group that did not get the procedure), four times as many clinical study participants were very satisfied with their night vision after the procedure. Pretty impressive, isn't it?

Sometimes the cornea is too thin to allow the removal of the flap containing the nerve endings, making LASIK impossible. An alternative method—called photorefractive keratectomy (PRK)—is used to reshape the cornea by shaving it down with a laser. PRK takes longer to heal and is more uncomfortable, because it does not lift off that sensitive flap, but the long-term outcome is the same as for LASIK.

When eyesight is beyond repair by LASIK and PRK, ophthalmologists can insert a phakic lens behind the cornea. (A phakic lens is essentially an extra lens inserted into the eye; the word *phakic* comes from *phakos,* the Greek word for "lens.") The surgeon makes an incision at the side of the cornea and inserts the lens either in front of or behind the iris. It is like having a contact lens inserted into your eye. The lens can be removed later if the prescription changes. In doctor talk, this is a prescription between –3 to –20 diopters (a unit of measurement for the power of a lens). I think I can safely bet that if you go from a –20 diopter prescription to normal in ten minutes, you'd use the word *ecstatic* a lot in your description of the change.

AMERICAN MEDICINE IS often criticized for the enormous amount spent on it relative to gross domestic product (GDP). LASIK surgery can cost $5,000. A phakic lens costs about $4,000. Inexpensive glasses can be made and distributed for $5 or less. You can wear glasses for the rest of your life; in fact, you can now buy glasses over the counter without visiting an optometrist. However, there is more to ophthalmology expenses than meets the eye.

The basis of the modern economy is knowledge. The number of patents a country produces is what puts that country on top of the economic scale—and the United States produces more patents per capita than any other country in the world. Advances like ocular procedures thus contribute to the nation's wealth. In ophthalmology, existing methods of treatment are likely to change every ten years. The benefits to such advances go far beyond the immediate benefit for the person receiving a particular procedure. Each new treatment adds to the knowledge base on which treatments for other diseases will be built; eventually, the number of patents will shoot the GDP high enough to eliminate disease. Furthermore, the patented technologies for vision correction and restoration are cost-effective, especially in light of what else we spend money on, such as televisions, cell phones, and so on. As with those electronic devices, the costs will come down as the technologies become more widespread.

Finally, what better use is there for our money than to spend it on the advance of medical knowledge? Is there something else we should buy instead of restoring and improving sight, especially for the 60 percent of sight- and hearing-impaired workers whose disability renders them unemployable?

RENEE MEJIA IS one of about 150,000 people living with keratoconus in the United States. *Kerato* means "cornea," and *conus* means "cone." A healthy cornea has a gentle curve, but when this membrane becomes loose and floppy, it can bulge out. The repeated trauma to the cornea from keratoconus makes the condition progressively worse. As a result of her weak, cone-shaped cornea, Renee had 20/400 vision; she had to be standing 20 feet away from a sign to read what a normal person can read at 400 feet away.

"You take a lot of things for granted with your vision," she says, "but it is no fun walking around a parking lot at night and not being able to find your car because you cannot see the cars. You don't know how frightening it is to be in a crowd trying to find someone and you can't see them. What is worse is that keratoconus gets worse over time. I did not really have the option of doing nothing if I wanted to be able to see."

Renee Mejia is 33 years old.

"I couldn't move where I lived because I had to be within 30 minutes of my job so I would not have to drive at night," she says.

"I did not change jobs for the same reason. I had to be close to home so I could drive only while it was light out."

"What was the worst part of your disease?" I ask. "What had the biggest emotional impact on you?"

Renee responds: "One time my partner slipped and fell on the ice and hurt herself badly. She hit her head. I couldn't drive her to the hospital. It was an emergency, and I felt helpless to take care of her. I had to stand there and wait while she was lying on the ground."

Renee's vision became so bad that she finally needed to have one of her corneas transplanted. Corneal transplantation, which has been around for a long time, requires a lengthy period of aftercare. The good news is that unlike a kidney or heart transplant, you do not need a lot of immunosuppressive drugs that make you vulnerable to infection. Sutures stay in place around the cornea for up to a year, during which the patient visits the doctor every few weeks to have a few sutures removed at a time. Remove them too soon, and the shape of the cornea becomes abnormal and so does the vision. It is slow to achieve the proper curvature of the cornea.

In 2004, the FDA approved a new option for Renee: the intrastromal corneal (or intracorneal) ring, manufactured under the brand name Intacs. The Intacs ring acts like a buttress that restores the normal shape of the original cornea and makes it stronger. The surgeon uses a laser to cut a channel into the cornea and inserts the ring. The natural outward pressure of the cornea closes up the gap and fits everything into place. The ring is a translucent, semicircular piece of plastic. It is barely visible, and can correct both astigmatism and refractive error. The procedure take 15 minutes and requires only topical anesthesia. The patient goes home the same day. The most important breakthrough is that it does this without the need for transplantation.

"As soon as I got off the table," Renee says, "I had instant relief. My vision went from 20/400 to normal in twenty minutes."

She can find her car. She can see faces in a crowd. She can move or change jobs without having to race home before darkness falls and the monsters come out. And most important, she is now able to take care of her loved ones.

Is this a reason to leap up and dance a jig? You bet it is. Every time I hear a senior physician talking about how medicine was better 25 years ago, I have to ask, "For whom?" Not for Renee Mejia.

She would have gone blind.

SHELDON FEINMAN IS a college professor who was going blind. Five years ago, Professor Feinman had a corneal transplant in one eye. Although it took a year of office visits and suture removal, eventually sight was restored in that eye. Professor Feinman is going blind in the other eye now.

Professor Feinman suffers from Fuchs' dystrophy, a weakening of the cornea to the point where, over time, it loses the ability to perceive and transmit light appropriately to the retina. In the last few years, a new procedure has been developed to give the same results as a corneal transplant, but ten times faster! The Descemet's membrane is the back layer of the cornea; it feeds, protects, and grows the translucent connective tissue above it. If you replace the Descemet's membrane on the inside part of the eye, it will regrow the cornea on top of it. It is like changing the soil in which a plant grows. After making an incision in the side of the cornea, the surgeon folds the new donor Descemet's membrane like a taco shell, slides it into place, and then unfolds it. A Descemet's membrane transplant—known as Descemet's stripping automated endothelial keratoplasty (DSAEK)—is 12 to 17 times faster than a normal corneal transplant.

Professor Feinman is the perfect person to describe the revolution: "Wham! There was really a tremendous difference. With DSAEK, I did not need stitches. I did not need to stay in the hospital. When I had the first transplant, it took a year to become normal. It was a year before I could drive. Now, after three or four weeks, I am nearly at normal vision. Also, I did not need to keep coming in to get the sutures removed . . . The outcome was the same in both, but now I got there in a fraction of the time."

MY FRIENDS THE OPHTHALMOLOGISTS are not as good as their patients at publicizing their advances. One day in morning report, around the time of my interviews with the Lazzaros, I talk about new advances in eye surgery like Descemet's membrane transplant and the phakic lens. I ask a room of 35 people how many of them have heard about the procedures, and only 5 hands go up.

A resident asks, "How come these people don't come up and tell us about these things?"

I can't answer. I also have to wonder how the general public can know about them when the residents in our own building don't. Even I didn't know about them until I sat down to talk with Doug and Clifford Lazzaro.

My investigation of ophthalmology is like surfing. The big kahuna is Doug Lazzaro. He takes me out on a beautiful day. We swim along nicely, then—"Paddle fast, here's the wave!" Migraine prevention, phakic lenses, Intacs rings, DSAEK. *Whoosh!* Man, is it exhilarating.

"And don't forget," says the big kahuna, "about riboflavin and ultraviolet light exposure to tighten up the cornea . . . You put a few drops of riboflavin, which is vitamin B2, on the eye. The riboflavin is given time to saturate the cornea. Then we expose it to ultraviolet light at the 370 nanometer wavelength. This will tighten up the collagen stroma of the cornea [the layer above the Descemet's membrane]. It makes the cornea stronger."

The procedure appears simple, safe, and easy to perform. It is an outpatient procedure, of course. It may stave off the progress of keratoconus for as long as five years and comes with an average improvement in prescription of two diopters.

"However," Doug says, "it is for keratoconus. It doesn't work for refractive errors."

I am struck by his disclaimer. What's next? "By the way Conrad, I cured cancer today, but it doesn't work for diabetes"? I'd rather hear Doug Lazzaro say, "Hey, today I restored sight to someone who would have been blind just a few years ago."

So much comes my way in the process of writing this book. In the symphonic orchestra of all the specialties of medicine, I am overwhelmed by the crescendo of human achievement. Not just eyes but ears, hearts, and minds restored. I feel the hope that we as a culture, a civilization, and a community will find all those cures that we seek. If we take the best of science and use it in service of a suffering humanity to relieve pain, then not only will we repair the damage to the body, but we will feel the kinship that makes our walk in this world together so satisfying. We will have an unprecedented ability to do good for one another.

I SHOW A DRAFT of this chapter to Doug Lazzaro, and he gets a big, 100 percent, light-up-Brooklyn look on his face.

"I do feel it, Conrad," he says. "I agree with you. I'm just not sure if I agree with you telling everyone that I am a guy who will paint his face at a ball game." To prove the point, he adds, "I took the kids to a Giants game last night, and I did not paint my face."

He laughs with the kind of good-natured warmth that puts patients completely at ease. His thinking is the polar opposite of the doctor-is-God mentality they tell me used to dominate the profession. Some doctors will look at your name tag, trying to note your position, before they talk to you. These people have one demeanor for superiors and another for people they consider further down the food chain. Doug is not like this. He is the kind of teacher we need training students to keep them from losing their humanity along the way.

PART 4

No Hope Is False

CHAPTER 13

The Danger of False Despair

False Despair Can Be Dangerous to your Health

A NDREW ROBINSON WAS 36 years old and at the peak of his powers. Outside of work, he enjoyed boxing, writing children's books, and studying his religion, Judaism. One day, on a vacation with his small daughter, he began to suffer from tiredness and a cough. Suspecting an infection, Andrew decided to stop off briefly at a local hospital for some antibiotics. A caregiver performed a complete blood count. A little while later, a physician introducing himself as an oncologist appeared. Andrew, an aggressive trial attorney with a take-charge attitude, knew to do three things: control the situation, learn everything, and don't trust doctors.

During my interview with him for this book, Andrew says, "A portion of my practice was medical malpractice cases. I have been on both sides of the fence. I was both a prosecutor and a defender in these cases, but in both roles, I was acutely aware of how things can go wrong in medicine. I can safely say that this only increased my level of fear at what goes on in the hospital. I was used to looking at medicine from the point of view of the mistakes that can happen."

Andrew tells me that his meeting with the oncologist went as follows: "Mr. Robinson," says the oncologist, "you have leukemia. It is very, very unusual for a man as young as you to have this form of cancer. Your white cell count is over 30,000, with the normal being less than 10,000. Normally people have ten to twelve years to live with this form of cancer, but you are anemic and your platelet count is low. In your case, the life expectancy is much less," I knew it might be as little as one to two years. The oncologist said, "You don't have to rush to go home. There isn't anything much that can be done about it, and you can finish your vacation. In any event, you will most likely be dead in five years. It is almost untreatable, and it is incurable. Good-bye."

Andrew adds, "I didn't even know what an oncologist was. Here I was given a death sentence in the bluntest way imaginable."

Physicians' narrow, "responsible" way of looking at things can have adverse effects on patients. It is understandable that we doctors are wary of offering false hope; however, we often go overboard and leave our patients feeling helpless and despondent at the very moment in their lives when they are in need of the strength that comes from help and hope.

Chronic lymphocytic leukemia (CLL) is a cancer of the bone marrow. For unclear reasons, a defect occurs in the development of white blood cells, which are in the business of making antibodies to neutralize infections. In CLL, the white blood cells fail to make antibodies appropriately. Infection enters the body, and the cells don't attack it. CLL is usually and almost exclusively a disease of patients above the age of 60.

Andrew continues to tell me the story of the year his life changed forever: "When I see the next oncologist, he tells me there are a few treatments such as fludarabine that can slow down the progress of the disease. He tells me there is a lot of research being done in the area. Although there is no cure now, he says, the treatments may give me enough time for something new to come that can save me. It turns out that the messages of both oncologists were *accurate*. Only the second one turned out to be the *truth*. The facts were the same in both messages. One rocked me with despair. One gave me hope."

I have known Andrew for over 20 years. For 15 of those years, I have been helping manage his care as one of the many physicians involved in the treatment of his chronic lymphocytic leukemia. Throughout this time, he has been telling me about how physicians deliver news, because I believe he knows I will deliver his message to a wider audience.

"If holding hands is not the duty of a doctor," he says, "then I don't know what else is. No matter what, patients need to feel that the doctor is there to help them. It is not the doctor's duty just to deliver news. Anyone can do that. The doctor's duty is to help them emotionally. Otherwise, what is the point? Then have an assistant deliver the news, write them a letter, send them a fax. You have to give doctors a dozen different ways of delivering news. They are all true. But one gives hope and the other gives despair."

During our discussions, I have to suppress my resentment at being lectured by a nonphysician on how physicians treat and speak to patients. Who is he to tell me what I already know? I have never dropped a death-sentence bombshell and then walked out of the room. I hope I am right. I wonder, though, whether one of my own patients is out there, somewhere, feeling angry and hurt by my insensitivity.

Andrew reminds me, "False despair is not so much what you say, but how you say it. Cold, distant, short, terrible news delivered badly. You have to be in touch with your own humanity first. You have to be vulnerable. Your patients may cry. Whether or not you can do anything for the disease, you can do something for their emotional outlook. If the news is bad, imagine how much worse it is if it's delivered badly. Tone is everything."

When I first started helping take care of Andrew, I was a fellow in infectious diseases at Memorial Sloan-Kettering Cancer Center. I helped treat some of the infections he developed at the time, but I did not think he would survive. Despite the fludarabine treatment, his white cell count continued to rise. When his counts rose to the ridiculous height of 400,000, I was mentally preparing to sit with Andrew and his family as I told him that his death was near and talked about ways to manage the end of his life.

In addition to Sloan-Kettering, Andrew hit all the major cancer centers in the United States: the Dana-Farber Cancer Institute in Boston, the M. D. Anderson Cancer Center in Houston, the Fred Hutchinson Cancer Research Center in Seattle. He left no stone unturned.

Andrew says to fellow patients: "You should never be hearing about anything new for the first time from your doctor. You should research everything beforehand on the Internet or with books. You must prepare to meet your doctor so you can discuss the options with him that you have already found out about. And remember, many people are afraid of asking the doctor questions that might upset him. That is also why it is important to take care of your doctor's feelings."

A staging system is the basis for determining severity and treatment of cancers. The staging system in CLL is the Rai staging system, named after Dr. Kanti Rai, who works at Long Island Jewish Medical Center. Early, or stage 0, disease requires no treatment, and you can live for over a decade with it. For advanced, or stage IV, disease such as Andrew's, you can expect to live only a year.

Andrew learned about the Rai staging system from a book. He figured it would be a good idea to go see the guy for whom the staging system was named. The result? He learned that the only things anyone could offer him, besides the fludarabine he'd already been taking, were medications to manage the infections: antibiotics and monthly infusions of intravenous immunoglobulins (antibodies produced by healthy white blood cells).

After his visit to Dr. Rai, I didn't hear from Andrew for a while. Then, out of the blue, I got a phone call from Israel. Andrew, not accepting the fact that no one in the United States would do a bone marrow transplant on him, had decided to leave the country. He had learned of a former Israeli commando, Professor Shimon Slavin, who might help him.

Professor Slavin carried out a bone marrow transplant for Andrew, with Andrew's sister as the donor. Months, or maybe only weeks before he was to die, Andrew was snatched from the jaws of death: the transplant was successful. No evidence of disease! That was over ten years ago. Andrew Robinson is still in a sustained remission—that's oncology-speak for *cured*. (Oncologists use the term *sustained remission* instead of *cured,* because they do not know what the future brings. They're afraid of commitment.)

Asked what the main thing is that he owes his extraordinary survival to, he says, "Depending on your worldview, it is either luck, fortune, or blessing."

"Come on, Andrew," I chide, "you have been incredibly proactive and aggressive in seeking out knowledge about your disease and traveling all over to get the best care. You do not seem to me to be a man waiting for 'luck, fortune, or blessing.'"

Andrew replies: "All people bring their worldview to their disease. Some people simply put themselves in the hands of their doctor. I have screwed up enough to feel that there is luck, fortune, and blessing."

Andrew's aggressive personality, hard work, and belief in "luck, fortune, or blessing" allowed him to survive long enough for research to catch up with what he needed: a cure. It's as if he'd been riding a train toward the end of the line and the track was being laid down even as the train hurtled forward.

Andrew now says, "We are living in the age of miracles. If I'd had this disease even a few years before, I would have been dead."

He tells me that Professor Slavin, a nonobservant Jew, once told him that it was good that he'd come to Jerusalem to be treated, because Jerusalem is closer to God.

ONE DAY, WHILE Andrew was recuperating in Israel, he and his wife suddenly heard a horrible sound.

"*Crack!* That's what I heard," Andrew says, "and what my wife was able to hear from the kitchen."

It was the sound of his spine fracturing. Bone marrow transplantation presents more than a few deadly problems. The recipient can reject the donated bone marrow, or the new immune system that comes with the donated marrow can attack the recipient. Physicians use powerful immunosuppressive medications, such as the steroid prednisone, to prevent these conditions. Prednisone is loaded with side effects, including osteoporosis (thinning of the bone). Essentially, steroids raise sugar (glucose) levels for the body to use in stressful situations. One of the ways they do this is by sucking the protein out of the bone to use it as a substrate for glucose formation. The bones, and muscles too, become sugar. Steroids can dissolve your gluteus maximus to form sugar for instant energy. Your ass really can be candy!

Andrew had developed such severe osteoporosis that the weight of his own body broke his back. The bone fragments put pressure on his motor and sensory nerves, and the pain was excruciating. For months afterward, Andrew was unable to sit up or walk. All he could do was wait for the problem to resolve spontaneously. His wife put him in a wheelchair, and he spent a lot time sitting outside in nature. A friend sent Andrew a camera and a telephoto lens, and Andrew became a nature photographer. Over the slow months of recovery, his pictures accumulated. On his return home, they made it into a photo exhibition in New York City. Some now line the walls of the Bone Marrow Transplant Unit at Brooklyn's Maimonides Medical Center to inspire patients, families, and physicians.

When I ask Andrew how he made it through his illness, he replies: "Engagement, no matter what it is. As long as you feels engaged with something that is important, whatever it is, as long as it provides meaning, purpose, and a sense of accomplishment, engagement will save you. It could be knitting, it could be going to a baseball game. It doesn't matter."

I wonder how much of Andrew's survival has been caught up with his tremendous "engagement" in trying to deliver his message on how to deliver messages: "The main thing that leads people to despair is how the news is delivered. In all my speaking with patients, I have never seen anyone given false hope. I have never heard of one patient given false hope, but I have heard of many patients given false despair."

A FEW MONTHS LATER, Andrew was walking again. He completed a book of ABCs for children using the paintings of Vincent van Gogh. His vision was bothering him. He avoided confronting this one; it was just too much. What now? Cataracts, another side effect of steroids. Left untreated, this milky clouding of the lens will blind you. Andrew opted for cataract surgery. After a 20-minute operation—*pop!*—his vision was restored. This is hardly a miracle to the surgeon, but to Andrew Robinson, a man who found his way out of pain and despair through photography and making illustrated books for children, that's exactly what it is.

I tell Andrew about the paradox of my profession, in which doctors are losing enthusiasm at the same time that we are able to do more than ever for patients. To heal more, cure more, relieve suffering more.

He says: "My feeling is that most doctors, the ones who are unhappy, have lost the sense of relationship with patients. The one-on-one, human relationship is missing, which is most satisfying. My doctors understand who I am. I know a lot about my illness. So you should understand as much as you can about your disease. You want a doctor who understands something about you." He says that he tells fellow patients, "It is important for you to take care of your doctor! When you meet doctors, tell them things about yourself as a person. Make yourself an individual to them. Tell them a joke. Make yourself distinct to the doctor. Ask them how their day is going."

A FEW YEARS after the transplant, Andrew, his family, and friends began to use the word *cured*. His back improved, his bones recalcified, and he got slowly better. Over time, however, mobility had become a problem. His knees hurt. Walking up a staircase was slow. Andrew's osteoporosis had progressed to the point where he had no knee joint.

"It was bone rubbing on bone," he says.

What a disaster! Cured of cancer, only to become disabled. Cataracts removed and sight restored, only not to be able to walk anywhere.

I saw Andrew a number of times during this period. Although his spirit stayed strong as ever, he became physically fragile. His shoulders thinned to the point of protruding bones. Everything stuck out. He kept a bag in hand with a cushion in it always. Even in an upholstered chair, he needed an extra cushion. His skin, partially discolored from his body's dealing with the attack of donor marrow, took on a sickly, translucent quality, with patches of old pigment. An ordinarily difficult walk down a hallway and up one flight of stairs took on a preternaturally prolonged discomfort. Not yet 50, the father of a young child, Andrew was unable to run, bike, or even move in a normal fashion. As a hyperkinetic person myself, always ten minutes late for everything, and always running, the slowness of his movement broke my heart. I had the urge to scoop him up and carry him.

One day while exiting a cab, his hand gripping the door for stability, Andrew crashed to the ground as the cabbie started to drive away with the door still open. Andrew was left lying on Broadway with a fractured pelvis and elbow. He knew that his immune system was severely compromised, so it took him some time to work up the resolve to undergo a major operative procedure. Andrew finally decided to get both his knees replaced.

When he told me, I smiled; it is my duty as a doctor to project confidence. However, I had known Andrew for such a long time that all I could see was a list of risks:

- Infection at the wound.
- Clots that fly up to his lungs and kill him.
- Blood thinners that make him bleed in his brain and in his guts.
- Failure of the artificial joints.
- Cardiac rhythm disorder during the procedure.

At times like this, I wonder if I really should be taking care of people that I start to feel too personally close to. Even though the risk of each of the things I stated is small, they ring out to me like the sound of a closing door on an airplane for a person with a fear of flying.

Andrew, however, had a different take on fear.

"Fear is a great motivator. Fear of death. Fear of not being prepared to visit the doctor. I knew where things could go wrong in a hospital, but I was also scared to do nothing. I knew that if I did not get my joints replaced, it would only get worse. Fear of it getting worse moved me," says Andrew.

The day after his knee replacements, I was walking toward Andrew's room at the Hospital for Special Surgery. My mind was a corkscrew on that beautiful day. Partly I was saucer-eyed at the elegance of this fantastic hospital and grateful to the people who donated the money to build it. My patient and I would never meet the donor, never thank him or her in person, never express our admiration for the building's clever design, despite the good done to me and him. But together with my awe, I dreaded what I would find in Andrew's room.

In a flash it all changed. Andrew was standing, taking a few steps between beds with the help of an aide. Little pain. Cracking jokes! Two days later, he walked out of the hospital on two brand-new pieces of polished titanium.

A month later he was dancing!

Fifteen years after his diagnosis was made, Andrew and I are sitting in the patient lounge of the Hospital for Special Surgery at Weill Cornell Medical College in New York City, doing the interview for this book. Andrew is recuperating after having a fractured hip repaired from a fall he took after being jostled on a crowded city street. We are talking about the miracle of the cure of his CLL by a bone marrow transplant. As I watch him settle into his chair and try to find a comfortable position, I am filled with gratitude and a feeling of immense luck. Just 24 hours after surgery to put a rod into his hip, this man is up, out of bed, and taking his first few steps. Here is a man whose spirit has been polished, melted, and reformed in the forge of immense suffering. Andrew tells me his wife and daughter will be joining him. He rejects my offer to reschedule around his family time.

His wife, Jill, starts things off by saying, "You never know what will happen. No one's life is set in stone. But we are compelled to live, we are compelled to live."

"What do you think is the most important factor that has made Andrew do so well?" I ask.

Jill responds: "He is surrounded by people who love him. We fail all the time and let each other down. Yet, you just can't survive alone when there is nothing to survive for."

"What would you do differently if you had it to do over again?" I ask.

"I would have gotten more help," Jill says. "I would have enlisted family and other people to help earlier. I couldn't even bring myself to hire a person to come to help in the house. Between a husband and wife, there has to be a certain formality, and certain distance."

While this conversation is going on, Andrew's daughter Leah is playing with her cell phone. I am annoyed that she is not paying attention. So, in characteristic subdued fashion, I force the issue. "Andrew, is there any one person who gives you a reason to live?"

"The people right here. Leah, Talia [another daughter], Jill."

"Do you think you would have given up without them?"

"Maybe."

Suddenly, I understand why Andrew wanted me to know that I would be doing this interview in the presence of Jill and Leah. Now I know why I am here. To help deliver a message: "I might not have survived without you."

Andrew is alive because of his aggressive stance toward conquering his disease—for his wife and children.

"Leah," I ask, "is there anything you think you have different in your relationship with your father because he is sick, that other girls don't have?"

"I just don't think of him as sick," she says.

"Do you see him as strong or as fragile?" I ask.

"Well, strong and fragile," she says. "His bones are fragile, but he is strong."

"What is strong about him?"

"Even when he is in pain, he is happy. Even though bad things are happening, he is still okay."

Jill interjects with her own question to Leah: "What do you think about your father having a chronic condition?"

"I don't know," Leah says. "I don't think of him as having a chronic condition."

Is she in denial? Insensitive? Blind? Ridiculously overly optimistic? No. Here is a daughter seeing her father through the lens of the strength and grandeur of his spirit, the purity and sweetness of his soul that has grown and developed because of this illness. Cancer: cured. Cataracts: cured. Broken, fractured: cured. Why shouldn't she see it as just another ordinary day?

CHAPTER 14

Only Connect

Hope and Empathy in Neurosurgery

A STORY:

One moist and uncomfortable night, Sir Percival comes to the castle of the Fisher King. The castle is in the middle of the Waste-lands. He is made welcome and led to take his rest in the middle of the great hall. In the middle of the night, a procession appears. A maiden appears with a spear that continually drips blood from the tip. This is the spear of the Roman soldier Longinus, which pierced the side of Christ as he was crucified. The rich Fisher King is placed on a couch at the front of the room clearly wounded, where he lies in great pain. Finally, a large platter covered with silk is brought in, held aloft by holy men singing praises to the most high. Percival perceives that as the Grail passes each table, all who sit are fed with that which they love the most.

Percival wants to speak but dares not. He sees the Fisher King, wounded and suffering, but remembers at Arthur's court the admonition to speak little, lest he reveal his poor education and look a fool to the other knights. Percival wants to ask "What ails thee, sire?" and "Whom does the Grail serve?" but he remains silent.

The next morning, Percival awakens with the castle gone and all that is visible a waste land. He rides and meets a holy man living in a hermitage. The hermit tells Percival that the Fisher King had been kept alive for many years by a single mass wafer brought to him daily by the Grail. He tells Percival that had he asked the question "What ails thee, sire?" the Fisher King would have been healed because of his compassion. Because of his fear of other men, Percival did not ask "Whom does the Grail serve?" which would have healed the Wasteland.

Percival begins his quest again on the road of penitence and faith.

It was a calm Saturday afternoon during my internship, and I was in the residents' lounge doing nothing in particular but feeling tired. It was far along enough in the year that the excitement and fear of starting training was over, but not far along enough to feel the end of training. Suddenly someone announced that a code was happening. A code is a superemergency. Codes are often labeled in the announcement so that you know immediately whether the emergency is a cardiac arrest, a seizure, a stroke, a fire, and so on. In any event, it means you are to drop what you are doing and run to get there. Only I didn't run.

The code was for a seizure on another floor. I wasn't particularly tired physically; I just didn't want to be bothered. I was focused on my own ease and not at all on the person with the seizure. I remember thinking something like, *Oh crap, another seizure,* then picking myself up, walking up the stairs, and stopping the man's seizure. I ordered the tests he needed: sodium, glucose, calcium, magnesium, a toxicology screen, and a CT scan of his head. I ordered the phenytoin (brand name, Dilantin) he would need to control the possibility of the next seizure. I did it all mechanically. No feeling. No compassion. There was no "person" for me who was seizing. There was just work to be done. A body in a bed. Synapses covered with bone and skin. Aberrant electrical activity possibly from metabolic abnormalities. My job only went as far as stopping the seizure and ordering the tests. I didn't care. I wrote a note in the chart: "Patient found with generalized tonic-clonic seizures. Diazepam 10 mg pushed with resolution of seizure. Tests ordered. Phenytoin started." I did not feel special or even good about doing the precise testing and treatment. I didn't feel anything except that my Saturday afternoon was interrupted by a problem to handle.

And yet it bothered me. A day or two later in a meeting with my teacher and a large group of colleagues, I brought up that I did not run to help the patient. I admitted that my first thoughts and feelings were about being inconvenienced. My question was simple: "What is wrong with me?" I expected some kind of reassurance, someone to tell me the situation wasn't serious (it was) or that I was tired (I wasn't) or that it would pass.

My teacher gave me a different response: "You are heartless, that is what you are, a heartless man. If you were in another profession, I might have a different response, but there is too much at stake. You are going to kill somebody through your action or inaction. But in any event, you should do something different. You should leave medicine. You shouldn't be a doctor. How could you ignore someone having a seizure?"

Her tone was matter-of-fact but firm. It wasn't harsh in the sense of being judgmental or angry or having any degree of personal dislike. It was an assessment. It was a measurement.

She continued: "If you don't feel the suffering of someone who is having a seizure and needs you, you need to leave before you hurt someone. Go do something different. You can find another way to pay off your student loans. You can't hurt someone." Then she made me an offer, sort of: "You can take a few months to try to do better, but I don't think it will make any difference. You should leave. I am sorry."

The event was life-changing for me. It was suddenly clear what I had to work on: empathy. Ever since that moment, I have been on a quest to be a man of great heart. I started out at the time to prove my teacher wrong. The more she challenged me, the harder I worked. She was right, and I knew it. Heartlessness was the only explanation for wrong circuitry in my emotional wiring. I strongly considered leaving medicine, because I did not want to be dangerous. But her response transformed me.

There is a tremendous power in knowing precisely what your problem is. I set out to change my character weakness into a strength. Over time, I began to develop the capacity to identify and even understand other people's suffering. Because I tried. I made efforts. I went back to the same professor over and over and over with various aspects of the same problem, and she helped me overcome my inability to recognize the pain of others.

Her voice of discipline still rings out to me through the years: "You are heartless. I want you to work on this and give me a very good reason why you should not leave medicine."

Years later, the same professor developed some medical problems. In the paradox of life, I became one of her doctors. Every once in a while, the subject of my heartlessness came up. It was never whitewashed, downplayed, or forgotten. She was as straightforward as ever: "You opposed me and set to work on your problem. You have grown. That is why you are so useful now."

When her husband became ill, I became the go-to guy for all serious decisions on his care with his regular doctors. When they were frustrated, they got me. When the system did not work, they got me. When he was in pain, they got me. And when her husband was at the point of death, I was brought across the country to be his personal physician and to accompany him in the private jet that flew him back to New York.

"Here's my samurai!" the man would say when he saw me. When he started to die in the back of an ambulance on the way from the airport, I used all I knew to keep him alive long enough to make it home, where he could depart from this world in peace, in the arms of the woman who loved him. The care of my professor and the man she loved for 30 years has been my most sacred act as a physician.

Over time, I believe I have become more empathetic, but at the core of it I still have the same problem. I first became aware of it 20 years ago, and I have been working on it ever since. The great ministers and priests may be right when they say that we preach what we need to hear.

I see an alarming number of unhappy or unsatisfied physicians today. If I bring up an advance, they bring up a weakness. If I bring up a new, highly effective therapy, they bring up a side effect. If I bring up new research, they bring up insufficient funding. If I bring up the fact that we are the highest-paid profession in the country, they bring up the cost of malpractice. If I bring up that the public trust of physicians is at an all-time high according Gallup polling data, they not only refuse to believe it but vigorously disagree. If I were to tell them they'd won a million dollars, they'd tell me they have to pay taxes on it. If I said they'd won a 50-room mansion, they'd tell me how hard it is to keep the rooms clean.

This negativity is alarming because a doctor's emotional health can have life-and-death implications for patients, as my apathy nearly did for the seizure victim so many years ago.

Throughout the hundreds of interviews I conduct for this project, I am surprised by how many patients will tell their stories over the phone to a man they have never met. It is true that their doctors have called them and told them I am a physician writing a book on hope, but still it is remarkable how people open up with even the slightest prompting. Perhaps it is because I can do something their regular doctors either can't do in the limited time span of an office visit or won't do because of lack of interest. For whatever reason, every single person I speak to is ready at any time to tell me anything I ask. Except M.L.

M.L. has suffered from epileptic seizures since the age of five. He does not want to talk to me over the phone about it.

I have been expecting something like this—the wall of privacy—but I am puzzled. I don't know of any social stigma attached to seizures. They could not possibly be viewed as a personal failure. They are not sexual in etiology. There is no illicit substance involved.

But the reason M.L. does not want to talk on the phone about his seizures turns out to be nothing like what I suspected. It's not about privacy; rather, M.L. wants so much for me to understand his story that he insists on seeing me in person.

He says, "I am used to telling my story, since I have Medicaid and see a new doctor in the clinic almost every time I come. Although I don't have a title, I function as an 'adjunct professor of medicine' because of all the students and residents I have taught about seizures over my lifetime."

Well, surprise, surprise.

He continues: "I have to stay poor enough to continue to qualify for Medicaid. I would like to make more, but as soon as I go up above a certain level, I would lose coverage but would have to pay six hundred dollars a month for my seizure medications. I am trapped. If I make no money, I have coverage but not enough to have the kind of life I want. If I make too much, I have a better life but not enough to cover my medications. I have no way to leap up to the kind of income that would allow me to buy my own health coverage and still be able to afford to live."

"What do the people who have to fork up six hundred dollars a month for medication do?" I ask.

"They go to Canada."

The reason M.L. does not want me to use his full name has nothing to do with privacy about his medical condition.

"I have to work off the books," he says, "and I don't want to get into trouble if that is discovered by the wrong people."

As forthcoming as people have been with me about their medical issues, they are private about economic issues.

M.L.'S MATTER-OF-FACT, unemotional tone could almost be taken as a sign of mental illness, except that he probably learned it from eminently sane doctors determined to offer him no false hope. He has had as many as four seizures a week, year after year.

"I have come to accept it," he says. "One minute you are walking around, and the next minute you wake up on the floor or on the street."

"Isn't that painful and frightening to you?" I ask, trying to imagine what it is like to have an instant intimate relationship with concrete. "Don't you hurt your head?"

He says flatly, "You get more back trauma, actually, or seat trauma. You bang your hands and you don't know why."

M.L. suffers from complex partial seizures, which are defined by physical movement of one part of the body accompanied by the loss of consciousness.

"In the year before I had my surgery," he says, "they kept getting worse. I was getting them every other day. I could feel them coming on because I got an aura beforehand."

Although he took multiple antiseizure medications, M.L. kept having seizures, which increased in frequency over time. There is no single universally effective medication for seizures, nor do doctors know which drug to prescribe first. Finding the right medication is a matter of trial and error.

Seizure management is paradoxical. The record of seizures is thousands of years old. There are mountains of scientific and clinical research published in journals whose entire contents are devoted to seizures. There are subspecialty fellowships in epilepsy. Doctors can precisely describe what seizures look like and have identified dozens of correctable and temporary causes. The electroencephalogram (EEG) gives a precise reading on the electrical patterns that occur, and there are over a dozen FDA-approved antiseizure medications. On the other hand, we are only two steps farther ahead than Hippocrates in knowing what causes epilepsy.

Epilepsy happens. Neurologists specializing in seizure disorders are some of the best-educated ignorant people I know. Do you feel reassured? I know you are waiting for the "miracle" part on this one. Me too.

"WHAT EMOTIONAL IMPACT has it had on you to have seizures like this all the time?" I ask.

"Not a lot," M.L. says.

Either I am missing something, or M.L. has a serious psychiatric disturbance. Why isn't he angry and fearful? The answer is that he has spent his whole life with the problem. At least, that is what he says.

"What is the most frightening thing about having seizures like this?" I ask.

"Driving your car when you know you shouldn't be driving, and wrecking your car and not remembering what the heck happened."

My eyes go wide with astonishment. "How often did that happen?"

He responds: "I shouldn't have been driving."

Persistent, I ask it again: "How often did that happen?"

"That happened two or three times. It's not that I didn't know I shouldn't be driving."

I feel sad for him, but the feeling is mixed with fear for society at large. Did you know that a physician does not have the legal right to remove the driver's license from a patient with a seizure disorder? It turns out M.L. is quite the pro in this area of medicolegal ethics. He sounds like the section out of my own textbook on medical ethics: No two states have the same rules. There is, amazingly, no mandatory requirement for the physician to report seizures to the state. There is no protection from a lawsuit if the physician does report and the patient sues the physician for harming his ability to work. There is no universal requirement for how long a patient has to be seizure free before he or she can return to driving.

"Seizures have a big effect on not being able to do certain types of work. It happened when I was working in an office too. I would just start to wander off . . . and then start seizing."

M.L. is not close to his family: "I was sent away to school at age thirteen," he says. "I was sent to Israel at age fifteen."

He is socially isolated. He lives alone. He is 38 years old, never married, childless. He does not have a romantic love relationship.

He says: "It has a big impact on your social life. "

"Aren't you lonely?" I blurt out. My profession allows me to intrude into people's emotional lives I hope.

"You get used to it," he says.

But he is lying, or at least minimizing the pain of his loneliness. It dawns on me that this is why he wanted to see me in person. He is starved for empathy. We spend over an hour together talking about everything. For a while, he is less lonely.

"I ask a lot of questions of doctors," he says. "It leaves me less trusting of doctors."

"Do you trust your doctor now?"

"Trust, but verify," he quips.

M.L.'S DOCTOR, ETHAN BENARDETE, a neurosurgeon at the University Hospital of Brooklyn, tells me about a new surgery to treat epilepsy: "In properly selected patients, two out of three patients can have their seizures controlled with this procedure. People still may stay on medications, but either they are seizure free or there is a marked reduction in the number of seizures they have."

As part of the procedure, he explains, the surgeon removes about three centimeters of the temporal lobe and the amygdala (a small structure in the brain linked with mental and emotional states).

"What goes with that? What do you lose?" I ask him.

"Nah! You don't miss it," he says.

"Are you kidding? You remove a few centimeters of brain and you don't miss it?" Silly me. All these years trying to improve my brain, and the neurosurgeon says I have a few centimeters to spare. "So, Ethan, what do you do with it? I mean, you don't bread it and fry it and eat it with a glass of Chianti do you?"

Ethan Benardete takes that as his cue to leave. He is a brain surgeon and sees that the goofballs in my brain are unresectable (impossible to remove surgically).

M.L. UNDERGOES BRAIN SURGERY.

From Dr. Benardete's operative report: "The patient is a 38-year-old, right-handed gentleman with a long history of medically refractory complex partial seizures. The patient has tried multiple regimens of anti-epileptic drugs without a satisfactory reduction in his seizures. M.L. has several seizures per month. We concluded that M.L. would be a candidate for right anterior temporal lobe resection with resection of the amygdala and hippocampus as well. We will attempt to reduce the number of seizures and also decrease the severity of the seizures."

Afterward, I ask M.L. how effective his surgery has been.

"It's too early to tell. It's only been a year."

"How often do you have the seizures since the surgery?"

"I don't actually have them anymore."

Why doesn't he sound happy when he says it? I don't know what to make of this. M.L. palms off his underreaction as "That's just me," but there is something deeper here. He needs time for his life to catch up, like someone who has been in prison for 30 years with the expectation of a life sentence. Now he has been reprieved and the prison door is open, only he doesn't know where to go or what to do. Eventually cured after years of suffering, M.L. continues to suffer from the depression encouraged by his doctors' commitment to "no false hope." Still, I'm disappointed that he can't feel the miraculous nature of this success.

He sees this and says: "I still take six hundred dollars a month of medications. I still don't have the kind of work I want. I still get the aura of the seizures. So what has changed?"

I ask M.L. to tell me more about the auras he still gets.

"I get the aura like the seizure will happen," he says, "but it does not happen. It gets stopped because the part of the brain that would transmit the seizure to the rest of the brain has been removed. I get the feeling like I will seize, but I don't lose consciousness. It's not actually interfering anymore. It gets stopped."

Many doctors tried many medications for years but could not cure M.L. A neurosurgeon laid hands on him, and the seizures stopped. The man has been cured.

Nationwide, visits to alternative and complementary medicine practitioners have been increasing at a rapid rate, despite the fact that allopathic (that is, regular or traditional) doctors are developing new, good stuff all the time, and medicine is doing better than ever in terms of effective treatment. Why is this happening? I suspect the answer is empathy. Understanding. The explosion in alternative medicine seems to be based on its practitioners' emotional availability, sense of warmth, and compassion. In a doctor's office, you may get the feeling that the doctor's schedule is more important than you. He may in some way make you feel like little more than a paramecium. There's a lack of empathy. Your feelings are not important. Your suffering and your story are not important. Your pain and fear are not important. There is something perceived as more empathetic in the alternative and complementary environment.

I am not a naturally empathic or compassionate person. I am a warrior by inclination. Let's fight! Let's win! I do not have a natural empathic feeling, and the idea of sharing M.L.'s soul-crushing loneliness scares me. I do, however, have an impulse to protect patients from pain, both physical and emotional. Even if I have a limited capacity to want to feel M.L.'s loneliness, I can at least acknowledge it by saying out loud, "That must be so lonely," and not looking stupid or false when I am doing it. Even a nonempathic, hot-tempered narcissist like me can be taught to express empathy. An Olympic-level talker, I can also learn to pause after questions to give people time to answer. When they do, I don't have to feel their pain; I just have to acknowledge it. And, interestingly enough, that acknowledgment makes me better able to share and alleviate that pain.

I SPEAK TO ANOTHER one of Dr. Benardete's patients, a married man named Ron who suffers from a rare disorder called trigeminal neuralgia. The word *trigeminal* means "threefold" and in this case refers to three branches: the top, middle, and bottom of your face. *Neuralgia* means "nerve pain." The trigeminal nerve has only one function: to detect sensation on your face.

Ron describes the first time it really hit him: "I was walking out of a movie theater and was going down the stairs. The pain in my face came on so suddenly, *bam!* And then I was on the sidewalk rolling around in pain."

Ron began to have his pain in July 2006.

"It was pretty mild at first," he says. "I thought I had a cavity, because it was a pain in the jaw, so I went to the dentist. It was a flicker of pain at first. I had fillings done, and then redone. Then the dentist said there wasn't a problem with my teeth. So he sent me to an oral surgeon. Eventually I got sent to a neurologist. It took six months before I was finally diagnosed with trigeminal neuralgia."

(Although trigeminal neuralgia is uncommon, anyone with even modest general medical experience should have known that pain of the face that is sharp and episodic might indicate trigeminal neuralgia. It's my responsibility to tattoo every student who comes near me with this sort of knowledge so that some sorry son of a bitch like Ron doesn't have to sit through six months of pain while unnecessarily getting his fillings redone.)

"When I saw a neurologist, I finally got the diagnosis," Ron says. "They started me on oxcarbazepine [a drug usually used for the treatment of epileptic seizures], and it worked pretty well for nearly a year. Then I got married a year later, and on my honeymoon it got much, much worse. I went on more and more medicine, and the pain kept escaping around the medication.

"I told my wife that I had to be strong and not let the pain ruin my life. I couldn't back down. I said I couldn't let the pain make me timid. When I said the word *timid*, the striking of my tongue on the back of my teeth with the *t* and *d* sounds brought me to my knees with pain. I was trying to not be timid, and the very saying of the word cut me down."

I ask if it kept him up at night.

"No," he answers. "Trigeminal neuralgia doesn't affect you at night unless your mouth is really active at night . . . The pain was induced by simple tongue movements. Certain words could be very painful for me. There were some times when just saying certain words would just bring me to my knees. Certain foods could also be painful, like peanuts that you had to pick out of your teeth with your tongue. I could not chew gum for years.

"I am a teacher, but I was not able to talk normally. At any moment, a certain word could devastate me.

"I would choose not to talk. I was very emotional. When I came in to have my evaluation for surgery, I was in tears in Dr. Benardete's office. I was not thinking clearly; I was very disturbed. I was very dependent on my wife to make decisions for me. I definitely succumbed to a lot of emotions. Chronic pain is very debilitating. It makes you afraid."

As the trigeminal nerve exits the face through a bony canal, it can be compressed by arteries and veins. A little miracle called magnetic resonance imaging (MRI) was able to clarify this in Ron's case. An MRI has enough detail to show how the vessel squeezes the nerve.

Here is the operative report from Dr. Benardete: "The sterno-cleidomastoid muscle was elevated. The trapezius was elevated off the skull. A burr hole was placed in the skull and the bone flap was passed off the field for safekeeping. Once the bone was eggshell thin, it was removed. The 8th and 9th cranial nerves were easily identified. Under the operating microscope, the trigeminal nerve was inspected and seen to be compressed by two blood vessels. The anterior inferior cerebellar artery and the superior cerebellar artery were compressing the trigeminal nerve. Both of these vessels were moved away from the nerve. Teflon was used to move the loop of the artery away from the trigeminal nerve and completely decompressed the nerve."

"Did the procedure help?" I ask, a little anxiously.

"I woke up from Dr. Benardete's procedure in absolutely no pain, and from the moment I woke up, I have not had a single incident or flicker of any kind of any pain. My response to his procedure has been one hundred percent. Cure."

But, like M.L., Ron is still afraid.

"I am so afraid it will come back," he says. "As a matter of fact, I am banking on it coming back. I have a pretty terrible fear. Even when you are not in pain, the fear of pain coming at any time is paralyzing."

I interrupt him and say, "Let me tell you something: by the time it comes back, if it comes back, we'll have new procedures for you. We'll have something new for you. Like your car, by the time that car wears out, we'll have a new one for you. Next year's model. I promise!"

He says, "I believe in medicine advancing. I have a lot of confidence in medicine."

But I know he is saying this more for himself to hear, rather than really believing it. I tell him again, "I promise you, we will have new things to help you by the time you need them."

Ron is having a type of posttraumatic stress disorder. He is not fully healed because fear is killing his mind. Am I offering Ron false hope? I don't believe so. One of the biggest errors a doctor can make is to let fact trump or, worse, trounce, feeling. Some of us go so far as to set up fact in opposition to feeling. We use "truth" like an anvil in a Road Runner cartoon. It can be overkill. Yes, Ron has had the most advanced procedure for the moment. But it is also true that advances are coming at an astonishing rate. In the hundreds of interviews I have conducted, not one person has said he or she was given false hope. I discuss with doctors the idea that a hopeful truth may be more important than a scientific one. They do not agree. They are on the lookout to squash false hope. In the process, they may be saving a patient's life at his or her spirit's expense.

Empathy means to feel with the other person. That means the absorption or a least perception of another person's experience. I recognize Ron's fear and respond: "I am telling you, Ron, advances in medicine are flooding into availability at an astonishing rate. Your doctor is a very smart man. I am sure we will have something new for you if you relapse at some point in the future."

He relaxes. He laughs and says, "Okay!" Smiles.

"What is the most hopeful thing about your experience?" I ask.

His answer: "That people like Dr. Benardete are willing to devote so much time and effort toward perfecting their technique to help people who really need it. This is one of those conditions that is very private and not so well known, and it can make you feel really isolated. Chronic pain is very debilitating in the long term. It can really change your whole personality. The torture of knowing you have a lifelong possibility of pain can make you very scared.

" . . . I think you're right. The thing that kept me from falling into despair was holding out on the trump card of knowing that the decompression surgery was there for me. I kept it in my pocket, as a reserve, so that if the medications did not all the way work, I would still have an option. Knowing there was an option is what kept me from becoming completely depressed."

I am not sure that I am more empathic and compassionate than I was 25 years ago when I entered medical school. But I was fortunate to have a teacher who showed me how to express concern. I can only hope that Ron feels at least heard, if not understood.

DOCTORS ARE DOING amazing things that would have been considered science fiction 20 years ago. They are offering multiple new treatments that would have required a biblical figure only recently. So why are physicians not feeling good? I have made a logical, persuasive argument for optimism. My goal is to persuade the medical community that we have done so much; let us absorb the energy and do so much more!

People in the profession feel like managers in a chain store. They can bring glory, joy, and hopefulness by transforming the pain in someone's life, as did Dr. Benardete in the operating room. If he had the deep sense of emotional satisfaction and receipt of energy that comes from performing a miracle in someone's life, I was not able to detect it. Was he satisfied? Yes. Was he amazingly energized and euphoric? No. Is he defective or a bad guy because he did not feel it? Of course not. Life is a feast, and he is on a diet.

Most patients I approached about this project readily agreed to be interviewed, and many seemed hungry to be heard, to have the ear of a doctor who was interested in the emotional aspect of their illness. I am not saying that I'm the only one to do this, but physicians do tend not to wear their hearts on their sleeves. I am one who learned to be empathetic, or at least try, by lucky accident; I was fortunate to have a teacher who steered me in the right direction.

There is no formal program in place to train empathetic doctors, no expectation that empathy is important. Doctors know that it is important to do the right thing medically, whereas they see empathy as a luxury item, the Moët & Chandon of care. However, today's residents—tomorrow's doctors—are, I believe, more empathetic at least in part because, with duty-hour limitations, they are not as tired. However, empathy may not come naturally to many residents. If we can't teach empathy, the actual feeling, we can teach how to express empathy. We do that now in many schools. We have courses where actors play patients and students at least learn the right words to say: "That must be so painful." "You must be so lonely." "That is very sad." Sometimes the feeling will follow. But even if the feeling does not follow, the patients can feel that their physicians care.

Empathy is difficult to practice, especially for physicians who encounter suffering every day. If educators can recognize that many people are not natural at it and it is hard to do, they could create an open, nonjudgmental environment for students to admit shortcomings and try harder. Teachers need to regularly say, out loud, that it is not enough to be a waiter who throws the steak on the table and walks off. The emotional care must be clearly pointed out as important, and students and residents be measured on it—not only for the patient's sake but for the physician's as well. In Arthurian legend, the Fisher King is not healed when Percival fails to express his empathy. It is sad for the Fisher King, but the even deeper tragedy is Percival's failure to act from his compassion.

CHAPTER 15

Under the Aegis of Hope

Retina Reattachment Restores Lost Sight

THE RETINA IS a unique biological membrane at the back of the eye that takes light and transforms it into chemical signals for transmission through the optic nerve to the visual cortex at the back of the brain. One of the most heartbreaking problems of the eye occurs when the retina detaches from its base. It is easy for ophthalmology patients and their loved ones to fall into despair, because treatments for retinal detachment are not guaranteed to work. Treatments do, however, exist—and that is cause for hope.

Trauma to the eye, cataract removal, myopia (nearsightedness), and diabetic retinopathy (a noninflammatory disorder of the retina seen in roughly 2 of 5 people with diabetes) all predispose a patient to retinal detachment. Myopia gives an abnormal shape to the eye and can put enough tension on the retina to pull it off. Diabetic retinopathy leaves scars that can cause enough tension to pull the retina off. Sometimes, retinal detachment just happens without a clear cause. The patient loses vision suddenly, as if a curtain is being pulled down over a window.

Josheila Crandall is an administrator in the Department of Medicine at SUNY Downstate. She controls millions of dollars in our annual budget and must go toe to toe with physicians who do not want to be controlled by a nonphysician. She hires, fires, and disciplines dozens of people in clerical and support positions. She has to criticize her own boss. She must put people out of their offices to make space. Sometimes they rise up against her like an angry horde. She holds firm. We make progress. *Unflappable* is a good word to describe Josheila.

Her husband, Bill Crandall, was already blind in one eye when the retina detached in the other.

Josheila remembers the intensity of her despair: "It was like six months of being hungry but you can't eat. When I speak about it now, it tears me up. I would wake up at night and look at my husband and think, *This is a proud man; what is he going to do if this doesn't get better?* He couldn't wash himself, he couldn't even drink a glass of water because he had to keep his head down so the retina would reattach. It destroyed simple things you take for granted. He couldn't bend or stoop or put on his shoes. He couldn't watch TV because he had to be facedown."

Bill says, "I had to lie on my stomach for months till I got numb from the pressure."

"It was like having a baby," Josheila told me. "He couldn't even put the drops in his own eyes. He couldn't put on his own underwear. I had to do that for him."

"How did it start?" I ask.

Josheila says, "He was minimizing his symptoms. He had to be the macho man, but he kept asking me to schedule office visits for him."

DR. RICHARD LOPEZ, Bill Crandall's ophthalmologist, was able to save Bill's sight by a procedure called macular hole surgery. The macula is the focal point of all vision in the retina; it is like a satellite dish focusing all it receivers on a single point so that it can be perceived. If the macula is torn and thus becomes detached from the back of the eye, light does not transmit to the optic nerve. Being able to operate through the hole in the macula, repairing the retina, is crucial to restoring vision.

Dr. Lopez explains what happened in Bill's case: "The retina tore away in that hole and needed to be fixed. If this had happened twenty years ago, when macular hole surgery did not exist, he would have gone blind. He had cryotherapy and laser and a gas bubble placed, but the most important thing was macular hole surgery." Macular hole surgery is the repair of a tear or rip in the part of the retina near the macula.

I ask Josheila what the postoperative visit to Dr. Lopez's office was like.

"We have known Dr. Lopez for twenty years," she says. "He looked in Bill's eye, and he was silent, just silent. I thought I was going to have a heart attack."

The warm and well-meaning Dr. Lopez had nary a hopeful, encouraging word.

Josheila continues: "We are the kind of people who think that just when you think things can't get any worse, they do. I was thinking about what it would be like if the surgery hadn't worked. He would be blind in that eye too. He would have to be led around." Josheila was in the depths of despair. "Then I realized what the silence meant to the doctor: it was like 'job well done.' He was admiring the result! To him, that silence was golden, but to me I nearly had a heart attack. I am sure I got ten more gray hairs while waiting for him to speak."

A silent doctor can be terrifically anxiety provoking for a patient.

"When he finally did speak," says Josheila, "I wanted to do cartwheels. I was like a kid getting toys at Christmas. I wanted to run out of the room. I cannot describe the relief."

"WHAT I LIKE best is the immediate gratification of helping patients right away," says Dr. Mohamed Hajee, a fellow in retinal surgery at SUNY Downstate. "If a patient has a retinal detachment, you can inject an expansile gas into the eye in the office. Later, you can reattach the retina with cryotherapy or laser. Expansile gas injection has been around for the last ten years or so."

Mohamed combines personal warmth and patient care with the investigation of a clinician-scientist. He came to ophthalmology with a degree in engineering.

"I wanted to combine my engineering background with medical treatment," he says. "Ophthalmology advancements are very rapid. We have new methods of care almost every six months."

Mohamed brings me to the ophthalmology clinic to show me all the wonderful toys he has. Stunning new devices are everywhere. He spends 20 minutes trying to explain just one for measuring the thickness of the retina. Here is a physician who will take his direct observation of patient needs, both physical and emotional, and go into the laboratory to investigate the next big thing.

Dr. Douglas Lazzaro, the chair of the ophthalmology department (see chapter 12), talks easily about Mohamed's accomplishments: "Did you know he is a leading national expert on retinal blood flow?" he asks me with pride.

I didn't know that, though I'm not surprised to hear it. But like any trainee, Mohamed is susceptible to the culture of "no false hope." When I ask him about the triumphant stopping of macular degeneration in its tracks, his immediate response is, "But it is expensive."

To be fair, he is right. Still, I wish his impulse had been to start with the option and the hope. He quickly sees my point, especially when he realizes that these incredible advances are why he got into the field in the first place.

He says, "VEGF inhibitors like ranibizumab are the coolest shit, but we do have other drugs that do the same thing at a fraction of the cost."

The aegis is Zeus's impenetrable breastplate. You cannot be harmed or injured when wearing it. To whom does Zeus give it? Ares, the god of war? No. Zeus gives the aegis to Athena, the goddess of wisdom. To protect him from negativity, I want Mohamed to wear the aegis of knowing that he is the best person ever to come out of his program and that being the best means he has more hope to offer than any physician who came before. He has learned everything that was known and done in the past, as well as everything new. I say this to every trainee. First, it is true. Second, it makes them happy. Third, if teachers let trainees know that they are the best to ever come out of a program, they get the idea that they are powerful. A resident who feels powerful and more knowledgeable than his predecessors can feel that he can conquer any problem.

RICARDO BIANCHI'S RETINA detached under the strain of his extreme myopia. He is a scientist with a Ph.D. in physiology. He is trying to understand precisely how seizures develop, which will lay the ground for a more precise way to control them. He is the kind of scientist who works buoyed by the hope of one day conquering a terrible disease. Ricardo and I see each other every once in a while and have children near the same age in the same Brooklyn neighborhood. His Italian accent always reminds me of my childhood with grandparents speaking Italian over candles aglow in empty one-gallon Chianti bottles. Every once in a while, I call him Richard just to hear him say, "Please, Conrad. Ricardo!"

Ricardo has undergone one of the many treatments for retinal reattachment, which are all based on the mechanical reapposition of the retina onto the back of the eye.

Dr. Eric Shrier explains: "We put three ports into the eye. One is a light source; the others are to do cutting, suturing, and cryotherapy."

In cryotherapy, just a touch of super-cold liquid nitrogen fuses tissue together. In difficult cases, if gas, laser, sutures, and cryotherapy cannot get the retina to go backward to touch the globe of the eye, then you can put a band around the eyeball to squeeze the orbit so that it will touch the retina. The band around the eye squeezes it smaller so that the sclera comes in contact with the retina. This allows it to reattach.

If you can't bring the retina to the globe, then bring the globe to the retina. Small retinal detachments can be managed with an injection of an expansile gas into the eye, which can be done in the office. Over several weeks, the gas bubble floats up to push the retina backward against the globe of the eye. Again, it is a matter of finding unique ways to push the retina closer to the sclera so that it will reattach. It takes three months for the gas bubble to be reabsorbed and go away. This delay in reabsorption is good in the sense that the effect is long lasting, but difficult in the sense that the patient must endure an uncomfortable position for months.

When Ricardo tells me in his Italian accent about the multiple laser treatments he needed to reattach his retina, I hear the voice of my godfather. Ricardo describes having a gas bubble injected into his eye and then sitting with his head down for weeks for the bubble to work.

"The toughest part is not knowing what the results of the surgery will be for months," he says.

The recovery from a retinal detachment is slow. You have to wait for the tissue to reattach. You have to hope. In Ricardo's case, it went very well, but there was a lot of anxiety in the interim.

Ricardo says, "The most frightening thing is thinking that I would not be able to produce."

I expected his biggest fear to be dependency on others or not being able to read, not an inability to make the next breakthrough. He surprises me again with his answer to the question "What was the most comforting thing?" I expect him to say something like "getting the sight back" or "the love of my family."

Instead Ricardo says, "Dr. Shrier and the other ophthalmologists do research in the lab near me. He is an in-house guy."

To Ricardo, it's all about his calling to science: the most frightening thing is to not be a functioning scientist, and the most relaxing thing is to be taken care of by another scientist.

So when I ask Ricardo what he would say to patients with the same problem, his answer is poignant in light of his scientific perspective: "There is hope. Do not despair."

Bravo, bello!

PART 5

Think "Quality of Life" Instead of "No Cure"

CHAPTER 16

Look Me in the Eye

Oculoplastics Restores Dignity

"REMOVING AN EYE used to be the lowest task on the totem pole for an ophthalmologist. It was the task assigned to first-year residents to take out an eye. It was not respected," says Dr. Monica Dweck, director of oculoplastics at SUNY Downstate.

To be sure, when I was in medical school in the 1980s, when all the cutting-edge stuff like a corneal transplant, cataract removal, or retinal reattachment proved unsuccessful or impossible, then enucleation—removing the eye—was the beginner's task. Enucleation seemed to represent the failure of ophthalmology. It was a procedure to be over and done with, so that we didn't have to keep the patient around to remind us of our failure.

Monica says the magic words: "Oculoplastics is a change in our way of thinking."

Oculoplastics is a specialty in ophthalmology that is devoted to the beautification and restoration of the appearance of an eye. Whether you have a congenital loss of the eye (one that is present at birth), experienced traumatic damage to the eye, or developed an abnormal growth of the eye, doctors like Monica are there to make sure that the world perceives your eye, your face—you—as intact and beautiful.

Monica herself is the epitome of style. She is clearly the most elegant physician I know of in the hospital. She has an innate nobility that transcends mere prettiness. And this is the work she does with patients.

She says: "We are paying much more attention to the quality of a patient's life than we used to. The way the eye is shaped affects not only how we look but how we are perceived, our relationships, how the world interacts with us. Therefore it affects our psychology—our minds and our emotions. When I am repairing an eye to make the person look 'whole,' I am also repairing that person's ability to feel whole. To feel a normal part of the society. To not feel apart, separate, or ostracized."

Monica and other open-minded physicians like her are leading a quiet but powerful revolution that is bringing what medicine can do into line with what is most important to patients. Even when best health is not an option, dignity is.

"In the past," she says, "an ocular prosthesis was simply a ball inside the socket. Now we have so much more to offer people. We have hydrogel implants that expand over time as they absorb moisture. They attach to the socket. In the past, the prosthesis would not even really fit in. It would be too loose, it would fall out. We have only recently transcended our old thinking from the time when the false eye popping out was something that would happen and we would just be scaring kids. Now the eye implant expands osmotically. This is why people with engineering backgrounds come into ophthalmology. Some children are born without an eye, or have an eye that is badly deformed. You have to put in an implant that will expand and put pressure on the orbit, on the socket. If the prosthesis does not put pressure on the inside of the socket, then the socket does not expand normally, and the entire side of the head or face will be small and deformed. We need the expanding eye to prevent deformity. There are people called ocularists whose entire jobs and careers are based on making these prostheses and making them lifelike. This is an actual specialty, like functional art."

At first I thought that Monica just had the best jewelry in the building. Now I know the real best jewelry for an oculoplastic surgeon is the adornment of the soul.

If Monica had believed her forebears when they insisted that medicine was better in the past, she would never be advocating this new thinking. People outside the profession may find this obvious, but what we need in medicine is heroic men and women to smash through old ideas of what is possible and what should be done. Slowly, more physicians are understanding the impact of an illness on the emotional life of the patient. This kind of doctor heals not just a person's body but also her interactions with family, friends, coworkers, and society at large.

Monica Dweck spends her life breaking through to the frontier of making a restored eye, a routine miracle. She builds her own life in medicine on the hopes and dreams of other human beings.

ANN MARIE PRESCOTT had an extra piece of fleshy tissue growing over her eye out of the corner near the tear duct, a growth called a pterygium. A pterygium usually happens from an irritation to the eye from trauma or infection and sometimes strikes at random.

"It is embarrassing," says Ann Marie, a pediatric patient care technician, "when people walk up to you and ask you what is wrong with your eye and say that it looks red and inflamed. I couldn't look at you and talk to you. I did not want people to see my eyes.

"People would think I had pinkeye because it was inflamed. They got worried about my working with the children. I did not need glasses, but the growth in my eye was getting really big. It was like a big scar that was red. People would ask if it was contagious. And it looked so ugly!"

A pterygium is rarely threatening to a person's sight, but it can be threatening to his or her sense of identity and peace of mind. And Ann Marie is right: it is just ugly.

Ann Marie underwent surgery to remove her pterygium. The diseased part of her eye was replaced with an amniotic membrane from the hospital's tissue bank. The revolution, the routine miracle, here is the use of the amnion, in addition to the existence of a tissue bank that you can get just about anything from. For about the 50th time since I started these interviews, I am knocked flat by some incredible advance in medical therapy, while the doctor speaks about it as if the hot dog guy at the corner, the traffic cop, and everyone else knows about it.

A few weeks later, Ann Marie was confidently looking parents and patients in the eye. Her life was transformed.

"It brought back my true personality," she says.

THE EGALITARIAN CHANGE in thought that Dr. Monica Dweck works for and that Ann Marie Prescott enjoys—the idea that all people deserve to confidently look their fellow citizens in the eye—is currently limited to patients whose insurance will pay for it. People with insurance and access are of one sort, and those without are lesser. Only universal access to care can solve this inequality problem. Monica and her peers are big-hearted, clever, and fearless enough to repair the ocular deformities that make people retreat from one another. I hope that we as a nation are big-hearted, clever, and fearless enough to support them.

CHAPTER 17

Life Salvage

Rehabilitation Medicine

"T HE MOST AMAZING thing is watching people come in the door in a wheelchair the first time, then the next time with a walker, then walking by themselves," says Megan, the receptionist at Progressive Orthotics & Prosthetics, a privately owned facility on Long Island. I am on a field trip to see the computerized leg (C-Leg), the biggest miracle of the last 40 years in rehabilitation medicine. Like many people in medicine, Megan sees routine miracles walking past her every day. But with just a little push, even a casual observer will notice that two million years of human evolution take place in a few days or weeks as an amputee goes from a wheelchair to standing.

ACCORDING TO DR. PAUL PIPIA, chair of rehabilitation medicine at SUNY Downstate, "Well, there's not a whole lot new in my area. It's pretty much the same as it has always been."

But within five minutes, he is showing me YouTube videos of amputees doing things that transport him into the bleacher seats of a baseball stadium.

"Look at that! Look at that!" he says, pointing to the double amputee riding a bike. Or, "Did you see that? He's able to go down stairs with one foot over the other instead of having to stop to put each foot side by side on the same step!"

I feel like Paul is telling me to watch a man on first base stealing second.

"Look! This guy is walking all over the place. You can take a person who could barely move with a standard hydraulic leg and change it to a C-Leg, and in an hour he is walking. I have seen that a bunch of times."

Even video cannot convey the sense of freedom and movement that must come to someone who once would have been wheelchair bound or hobbling around on crutches but is now tooling down the street on a bike. What greater grace can there be than to be the inventor of such a device? Even so, if I were the amputee, I really wouldn't care if the greediest son of a bitch in the world made a computerized prosthetic leg for me with no loftier ambition than to be a billionaire. He gets rich. I get freedom.

THERE WERE 75,000 amputations in the United States in 2008 just from diabetes. This is actually down from a peak of 84,000 in 1997. In total, there are nearly 200,000 amputations a year in the United States, many of which involve young people injured in motor vehicle accidents.

Dr. Paul Pipia says, "I don't know what you feel about the war, but the best stuff is available from the government for amputees created by the war. The government put out a grant for research on prosthetics for amputees from the war. It does bring me some comfort that some good is coming from this troubling event." Paul adds, "Myoelectric is coming—there are devices, but they are heavy and don't work as well as we want yet, but they are close to being ready."

Myoelectric means that the prosthetic device senses electrical impulses from the nerves of the arm. The amputee's brain sends the normal impulse to the nerves. The artificial arm has receptors that pick this up and create movement. These impulses get transmitted into actual motor function in the arm. The arm can contract the hand and rotate the forearm.

"It won't be long," Paul says. "Right now, the response time of the myoelectric limb is slow. On the other hand, we already have a limb that can sense temperature. If you are a mother and want to tell if bathwater is too hot for your child to be put in, the artificial limb can sense the temperature."

Amputees can take some degree of hope from knowing that great things are just around the corner. I take some happiness in reporting that myoelectrically stimulated arms and artificial hands that can sense temperature are just on the cusp of availability. I believe that people can bear almost anything as long as they know that the suffering is temporary and that their suffering is not wasted. "People are dying, Alfred. What would you have me do?" Bruce Wayne asks Alfred the butler in the movie *The Dark Knight.* "Endure, Master Wayne!" Alfred replies. Seriously. Myoelectric is the biggest thing, and it is now.

AS WORLD WAR II came to a close, the United States and Russia divvied up between them not only German territory but also German scientists; during this process, an American officer covertly marked the files of the best picks with a paper clip. Hans Mauch, who had developed German weaponry during the war, was one of hundreds of scientists snapped up by the U.S. military in Project Paperclip to work for the U.S. Air Force. In his spare time in his Dayton, Ohio, basement, Mauch developed a version of aircraft hydraulics to create the hydraulic knee control system, the most widely used prosthetic for most of the last 50 years.

By 1957, Mauch had switched out of military work and founded Mauch Laboratories to work on prosthetics. Mauch devices are still used by hundreds of thousands of people. Mauch later combined his work with studies done by the Veterans Administration to create devices that remained essentially unchanged for decades. Mauch was also involved in the creation of a reading machine for the blind and an early version of the space suit. Who would have imagined that one of the brains behind a onetime U.S. enemy would do so much to help disabled American veterans?

The C-Leg is to the Mauch hydraulic limb as a color television is to black-and-white TV. The C-Leg "knows" where it is in space. It knows if it is in front of or behind the wearer. It is programmed via a laptop with a computer cable. With a click of the remote, the wearer can change the mode of operation of one of his body parts! The C-Leg can be set to sense the motion of walking with precise programming for weight, location, toe and heel pressure, and rigidity of the knee. When the wearer needs it to swing freely in order to do something like ride a bike, he pushes a button and, *click!*, the leg is free.

The pylon of the device, which attaches to the artificial foot, has sensing devices. Between 50 and 100 times per second, the sensors collect information on the location of the foot, the pressure being placed on it, and how much swing of the foot is desired. You walk more freely with the C-Leg because it is sensing how you walk and is adjusted for your weight. The standard Mauch leg does not sense pressure or make adjustments. When the wearer goes to bed at night, he takes the C-Leg off and plugs it in. It has the same lithium batteries as a cell phone and holds a charge for more than 30 hours.

You cannot walk down stairs like a normal person with the hydraulic leg, whereas with a C-Leg you can walk leg over leg. Paul Pipia also points out: "The 'energy requirement' for walking with a hydraulic knee joint for an above-knee amputation is usually about 120 percent above that of normal walking. With standard prostheses on both sides, you needed to exert 240 percent more effort than normal. If you were a debilitated or weakened person, you would have been stuck with being in a wheelchair because of that level of energy requirement. With the C-Leg, you don't need to exert yourself that much. That's amazing!"

The C-Leg does have its limits. Running is not recommended. The prosthetic leg is, after all, a highly sophisticated piece of computer equipment. The wearer can't swim with it, either.

"It would be like throwing your laptop into the water," says one user. "I use a standard Mauch hydraulic leg as my 'water leg' when I water-ski."

DANIEL BASTIAN SITS down with me to discuss the C-Legs that he fits people with at Progressive Orthotics & Prosthetics. Dan is a tall, robust 43-year-old man. I don't often meet other men above six foot three. He looks like he can drop to the ground at any moment and gut out 50 push-ups. Dan's office is a small museum of sports memorabilia. There are pictures of Yogi Berra, other Yankees players, and football teams. There's a collection of baseballs in a candy dish. All around there are also pictures of him, his kids, and a lovely woman he identifies as his wife. And there are toy swords and costume swords. He sees me looking.

"I am getting ready for Halloween with the kids. I go as a pirate," he explains.

It is only October 10, and he is already preparing himself for one of the biggest days on the kid holiday calendar.

He hands me a C-Leg. It is sleek and powerful, like a piece of technology in a science-fiction movie. Switched on, it makes a slight whirring sound.

"That's the sensors looking for input," Paul says. "The sensors scan fifty times a second looking for data on how to adjust the movement. I'll take you back and show you how it is programmed."

I wait for Arnold Schwarzenegger to come into the room as the Terminator.

There are pictures of Dan water-skiing and downhill skiing. The previous winter, I had made my own first runs down the bunny slopes; it took me three hours to do it without a crash to the ground. I felt quite mediocre as eight-year-olds whizzed past. Waterskiing I gave up after my first try, when I was dragged facedown in the water and tried to inhale an upstate lake. Dan clearly outclasses me in the manly-man-sports category.

In his pictures, only one leg is visible. Suddenly I realize that the C-Leg Dan will show me is very special indeed. Dan pulls up his pant leg. This is simultaneous with me realizing that the reason I can't see his other leg in the pictures: he doesn't have one. Dan is an amputee. He shows me his own C-Leg.

"I had my leg amputated eighteen years ago. It was the best decision my wife and I ever made," says Dan.

I think, *Well, how often am I going to hear a statement like that?*

Dan had osteosarcoma (bone cancer) of the end of his femur (thigh bone) when he was 15. He had dozens of operations to salvage his leg. This was 30 years ago. It is a miracle he is simply alive.

"I was told I would have six months to live," he says. "I had surgery and chemotherapy at Sloan-Kettering Cancer Center. I was an active kid. I played varsity football and basketball. Then I had to stop everything. Now I coach my son's baseball team and football team."

Now all the sports stuff around the room makes total sense. And the picture of the golf team with a caption reading "Four guys, five legs, no problems." There is nothing like a picture of four men in golf shorts with their single and double artificial legs visible that will drive the point home.

"What made you decide to have the leg amputated?" I ask, grateful that my biggest decision that day would be what to have for lunch.

"I had so many operations and needed so much care that my wife was becoming my nurse," Dan says. "I had the amputation two years into my marriage, and I have been married for twenty years now. I am sure that if it kept going on, we would have ended up divorced.

"I was constantly in the hospital. I was constantly in pain . . . I was living on Percocet."

"I waited ten years before I got an amputation—ten years and eighteen operations, and then I decided to get the amputation. Then my doctor called me a quitter."

You can imagine how it would sit with a fiercely athletic man like Dan to be called a quitter by anyone.

"My doctor eventually called me back and said that he would do the amputation," Dan says. "I told him I was going to have the amputation done but that he was not going to be the one doing it, because I wasn't going to have someone do a procedure he didn't believe in."

Dan continues: "In many cases, amputation is life-salvaging. Vascular surgeons are concerned about limb salvage, but I am concerned about life salvage. If I hadn't had my leg amputated, I wouldn't be able to do anything I am able to do now. It's a hard topic to bring up with a vascular surgeon. I don't want to offend them. I wouldn't have the ability to work out. I wouldn't be able to go fishing. I wouldn't be able to go kayaking.

"Besides the physical things, there were the mental things, of me being constantly sick, constantly in the hospital, constantly having to depend on other people."

We know that pain and disability can create agoraphobia. Disability narrows a person's life. You don't feel like participating as much. If you are a parent, you don't feel as able to be a parent as much because of less mobility. With disability can come depression, social withdrawal, and hopelessness.

Dan shifts the focus from his own story to that of his patients at Progressive Orthotics & Prosthetics: "My biggest problem with doctors—and we deal with a lot of vascular surgeons—is that they will look at amputation as a failure, a personal failure. They were not able to save the limb. They will allow some patients to go through seven small amputations and years in a wheelchair to allow an ulcer to heal. They view a [transmetatarsal] amputation as a success if they get the leg to stay on for six more months. Well, that person was not able to walk for that time. His body is debilitating during that time. Eventually he gets an amputation, and there will be some success with a prosthesis, but not as much as there would have been if the doctor had done an amputation earlier and allowed the patient to get used to a prosthesis while he was stronger. There is so much invested in hyperbasic chambers and wound care centers, which can be important—you have to give it a shot—but I think some people would have had better success with a prosthetic if they had just had the amputation and gotten used to the prosthetic."

I must admit that I have been exactly the type of doctor Dan is talking about. Dan's explanation is revolutionary for me.

IT IS A LITTLE JARRING, even for a doctor, when a man lifts his pant leg to reveal the port where his limb plugs in at night.

"My stump is very short," Dan says. "I only have a few inches of femur below the hip to work with." He then explains, "I had a skiing accident a few years ago in which I shattered my leg and had to have about eight inches taken off."

Will nothing stand in this man's way? He also floors me by saying, matter-of-factly, that he had open-heart surgery. Dan had a hole in his heart that was found incidentally for an insurance physical.

"I was six months away from having a stroke," he says.

Here is the veteran of dozens of procedures on his leg, amputation, accident, more amputation, and open-heart surgery. It prompts me to ask him what he is most grateful for.

"I am fortunate to have a business in which I can help someone else. So many people have given me so much in my life."

Dan suddenly starts to get up and turn. He becomes very emotional, and I see something wet start to happen near his eyes.

He says, "Let's go outside," and turns away before I can see too much. He continues, "So much from my wife, my parents, my brothers and sisters. I am one of nine children."

There it is. Gratitude in the attitude. At the end of it all, there is not the slightest sense of resentment or victimization.

When new amputees come to see Dan, they are dealing with not just the loss of mobility but also the loss of life as they knew it. Dan Bastian understands their fear and helps them cope with both losses. The loss of the physical mobility as well as their psychological immobility. His can-do attitude is clear as he shows me around the workshop in the back where he and his coworkers construct orthotics for patients.

"When I see patients at the hospital," he says, "they have no idea what life will be like. That is their biggest fear, the fear of the unknown. They don't know what their life is going to be. The great thing here too is that they come in a wheelchair, and they can walk out. After you give them a new foot, you are giving them their life back. They think their life is over. They have lost their leg. They have been debilitated for maybe over a year trying to get an ulcer to heal. They finally get an amputation, they think *That's it;* they think their life is over. It is far from that." He is his own best example: "After I got the amputation, I could go back to all the things I loved to do. I got back into competitive downhill skiing. My original degree was in computer science. I was working for IBM, and it was a great job, but I decided to get a degree in making prostheses, and I quit IBM."

I myself once aspired to be an Olympic fencer. I trained every day for hours for ten years. One day I discovered a Purple Heart pinned on a bulletin board in my fencing instructor's office, the first indication I'd ever seen of his service in Vietnam. "Wow! You must be a brave man!" I exclaimed, with the enthusiasm of an ambitious yet fearful 17-year-old. He responded: "The only difference between a brave man and a coward is that the brave man panics forward." He taught me to accept fear as part of the human condition. Heroes and brave people are not fearless. It's okay to be scared. What matters is what you do with your fear. Knowing that changed my life. Bravery to me became right action in the face of fear. To some people, I seem like a bulldozer. When in doubt, panic forward. When in doubt, choose action.

"What do you think allows people to adapt to their amputation the most?" I ask Dan.

"Mind-set," Dan answers clearly. "Desire."

He is speaking from experience.

Dan says: "When I meet new patients, I tell them—every one of them — 'Ninety percent of it is in your head. If you will and desire to do it, you will do it. It doesn't matter what anyone says.' I had a patient who was a bilateral below-knee amputation in a rehabilitation facility. They said he would never walk. He was on dialysis. He was very debilitated. He wanted to walk. When there, he never progressed past a walker. I said, 'You've got to give him a shot.' After he was discharged, he would come here, and he would walk in. He wasn't in a wheelchair. He did far better than they ever thought he would . . .

"Then there are those few patients that just give up. Ninety percent of it is mental. I can make you the greatest leg in the world, and it can sit in the corner. It's not doing anyone any good. I don't sugar coat it and tell them it will be easy. You have to work. While they are sitting in a wheelchair waiting for an ulcer to heal that won't heal, their body is debilitating. Even a week or two in the hospital off your feet can weaken your leg a lot. And it does not bounce back as fast as it debilitated.

"I had a patient who was a member of Delta Force who was shot down in a Black Hawk helicopter in Somalia like they showed in the movie *Black Hawk Down*. He was fitted with a leg here and reenlisted."

I didn't know someone could reenlist as an amputee.

Dan explains, "He had to complete a twenty-mile qualifying run with a full pack as an above-knee amputee."

Dan believes that social attitudes toward the disabled have evolved dramatically, but they still have a long way to go. "People still have no idea of what these people can do"

I mention Oscar Pistorius, the South African sprinter disqualified for the 2008 Summer Games by the International Olympic Committee because the bounce from his prosthetic blades and the reduced lactic acid buildup in his limbs allowed him to use less energy than a non-disabled runner.

It is an amazing paradox that an amputee athlete was disqualified from the Olympics on the basis that his prostheses gave him an unfair advantage, but Dan does not share my enthusiasm. "After all," he says, "if being an amputee is an advantage, then you would have athletes cutting off their legs to do better."

Still, he feels the disabled are an underutilized resource in American society.

"The possibilities are up to the patient now," he says. "Amputees are not being limited anymore in what they can do. The only limiting factor is themselves."

I see a picture on the wall of Dan in Halloween pirate garb. Sword, skull and crossbones, and a real peg leg. Dan as a dad without limits, the coolest pirate his kids will ever see.

CHAPTER 18

Diabetics Take Control

DIABETES IS ONE of the most ancient diseases on record. In the fourth century BCE, the Greek physician Hippocrates extensively described urine output and urine quality. The ancient Greeks called it *diabetes mellitus,* which means, roughly, "honey-sweet fountain." Diabetes is the body's failure to regulate blood sugar, or glucose, due to a lack of insulin, which cells require to pick up the glucose they need. It occurs when the pancreas fails to make insulin. Too much glucose damages the thin lining of blood vessels that feed every organ at the microscopic level. The damage clogs the vessels, starving the organ. Choking off the blood supply can lead to blindness, stroke, and death. Low blood sugar, or hypoglycemia, can make you light-headed or woozy, even to the point where you pass out.

It took about 2,400 years after the time of Hippocrates for researchers to develop the first effective therapy. The entire management of diabetes is now based on accurate measurement and control of glucose levels. Glucose control is like fencing, in which a properly held sword can save your life and an incorrect grip can kill you. "Hold the sword like a bird in the hand," writes novelist Rafael Sabatini in the adventure *Scaramouche.* "Not so tightly you will crush it, not so lightly that you let it fly away."

In 1921, Canadian researchers Frederick G. Banting and Charles H. Best derived insulin from a dog pancreas; in 1922, they saw its first successful use in a 14-year-old boy. The first oral agent to lower blood sugar was discovered by accident in 1942, when scientists experimenting with sulfa drugs as antibiotics noticed that a certain compound lowered the blood sugar in animals. More medications have been discovered by accident than by design. It took 12 years for the first oral hypoglycemic agent, chlorpropamide, to be approved.

Today the U.S. Food and Drug Administration has approved over a dozen types of insulin, but the method of administering insulin by multiple subcutaneous (under the skin) injections has not fundamentally changed. A person with diabetes may have to check her sugar as many as three to five times a day by sticking herself with a needle and testing a drop of blood. Every single day.

In my worst nightmares, an interrogator shines a hot light in my eye and threatens, "So you won't talk, will you, Conrad? Well, we have ways of making you talk! Stick yourself with a small needle." What do I care? The needle is small, and I am a strong man, six foot four. He can tell what I'm thinking and says, "Right, you won't break with the first or second or seventeenth needle stick, but after the five-hundredth you will tell us anything we want to know!" Suddenly I get nervous. After three to five sticks a day, multiplied by my entire life, I might indeed break.

DR. AGNES GLIWA is the director of the fellowship in endocrinology at the State University of New York at Brooklyn. At the top of her list of recent accomplishments in the discipline is a pocket-sized insulin pump. A plastic tube carries insulin from the pump to the other end of the catheter, which is implanted under the skin. The implant is not deep, and the patient changes the site every few days. The pump is set to administer a predetermined amount of insulin. It automatically squirts insulin into the diabetic every few hours, so she doesn't have to stop several times a day to do it herself. If the diabetic eats more than usual, she taps in the calorie count, and the pump injects extra insulin. If she exercises, she programs that in, and the pump decreases the amount of the insulin (an exercising muscle will pick up sugar without insulin). If the diabetic doesn't eat, she programs that in, and the pump will hold the insulin so her blood sugar doesn't go too low. In short, the insulin pump is the most advanced technology to deliver the most precise amount of insulin the patient needs to stay balanced.

There is also a device that can be implanted under the skin and feeds glucose information into a tiny computer that fits in the patient's pocket. Dr. Agnes Gliwa describes it as the size of a beeper or an iPod: "The device is smart. It records all the readings, will give a numerical and graphic readout with a linear graph, and is much, much more comfortable than injections."

The technology exists to add a glucose sensor to the pump in a completely self-contained system that would automatically administer insulin based on the sensor's reading. Amazing—and no more multiple needlesticks! You just change the site of the implants and refill the pump every couple of days.

"So, Agnes, why doesn't every diabetic have a continuous-readout glucose monitoring device?" I ask.

"Because they are expensive to buy and cost $350 a month to maintain if you include the cost of all the pieces."

"So what? We do a lot of other things that are more expensive."

"Yes, Conrad, but the insurance will not pay for it," she says.

I have experienced lot of joy and excitement from learning about medical advances, and a tremendous amount of anger and frustration that they are not available to everyone. Diabetes treatments are a top case in point. The disease occurs at a rate of 10,000 new cases a week—minimum. We deny hundreds of thousands of Americans the most accurate methods for managing glucose, even as we know that tight control of blood sugar prevents blindness, stroke, heart attack, erectile dysfunction, and kidney failure. Inadequate health insurance coverage and decreases in funding for research effectively allow diabetes to maim and kill U.S. citizens. We have enormous reason to be optimistic with regard to diabetes. The number of new medications exploding into development is amazing. If we all smack our legislators in the head hard enough, maybe there will even be enough research to result in a cure.

In all, I ask five endocrinologists what they consider to be major recent advances. Agnes Gliwa is the only one to list the insulin pump. It is the first thing out of her mouth. Agnes is the youngest member of the division of endocrinology, the least experienced, and the newest out of her fellowship. When I ask the other four doctors why they don't bring up the insulin pump, they all give me a sort of "Oh, yeah—well, I suppose so—not really" kind of response.

I surmise at this point that the youngest member of the division may simply not have enough experience to know the most important advance, so I speak to patients to try to get a bigger picture.

Lorraine Brooks is SUNY Downstate's go-to person for hospital staff to report unfair treatment. She fights powerful people in standing up for others. She is 56 years old and has been diabetic for over 25 years.

Lorraine starts the conversation by saying, "The insulin pump is the best thing that has happened to me since the time I found out I was diabetic."

Wow! Score one for Agnes!

Lorraine continues, "The insulin pump allows me freedom . . . I don't have to stop to run into a bathroom to inject more insulin. I don't have to inject myself over and over again. You have no idea what it is like . . . You have no idea what a burden it is. What a fear it is. What a pain in the ass it is to worry about your sugar all day long.

"In the back of my mind is always the thought *What is going to happen?* Imagine being in your car and being stuck in traffic. Maybe I will pass out if the sugar goes too low. If there is traffic at a tunnel, what if I get stuck without something to eat? What if I get a flat tire? You have no idea how much keeping your sugar under control dominates your life. If you have experienced an episode of low sugar, as I have—with shaking, sweating, and feeling 'loopy' or light-headed—you would understand the fear.

"I am going through menopause right now, and sometimes I get hot flashes. Before the pump, I had no idea if the symptoms I was feeling were just my menopause or whether my sugar was going low. The symptoms can be the same. It's frightening, and it is embarrassing."

Frightening I can imagine, but embarrassing? For a professional protective bulldog like Lorraine?

I had recently commented to an AIDS patient of mine that the death rate from AIDS had dropped so much that HIV infection had become just another chronic manageable disease.

The patient became very upset and told me, "You are *so* wrong! You have no idea. You have no clue. If I had diabetes, I could go out on the street and tell anyone that I had diabetes. You have no idea of the shame and the stigma and the embarrassment of AIDS."

So I am taken aback by what Lorraine says, and have to ask, "In what way is diabetes embarrassing?"

Her reply: "It is hard to be out with friends when everyone is eating, drinking, and carrying on, and you have to tell people you are feeling hypoglycemic. I was embarrassed, I felt weird, I felt 'less than' compared to others. No one else had to deal with it. I always had to think, *What am I eating? What is my sugar?*

"People would say things like 'Don't be upset, there's nothing to be ashamed of. Be grateful you still have your eyesight and your feet still attached to your body.' Although I could appreciate that, it did not take away the fear and the anxiety that I had. I know there are people who are blind. I know all of that, but that doesn't mean I am not scared.

"For the first ten or fifteen years that I had diabetes, I kept trying to get people to understand what it was like, and no one really got it. This included my physician. After a few years, I started to take control. I started to educate myself, and I started to ask questions. My doctor did not appreciate that. He got patronizing and told me, 'Why do you need to know that? Don't worry about that. I will take care of it.' He did not like me when I started to ask questions. After ten years, I changed my doctor. I only recently got the pump. It is has given me the freedom to not be so hypervigilant about my sugar. It is total freedom. I used to run to my glucose meter ten times a day when I got into menopause. I was constantly making myself crazy. Now I am free. Now I feel I am in control, and I am not at the mercy of my disease. I feel relaxed."

I TALK TO two more patients to cross-check what Lorraine has shared with me. They also use words like *freedom, accuracy, less discomfort,* and *relaxed.*

Lynnette Bagot is a woman in her midfifties who has been diabetic for over 20 years.

"I came in to have a baby, and they told me I was diabetic," she says. "When you don't know what diabetes is, at the beginning it is like a death sentence. When you have to inject insulin, you have to rotate the sites of the injections. The injection sites become hard. You get track marks. It hurts. It is not convenient. You have to run to the bathroom. If you are out, it is really difficult. I wasn't checking my sugar like I should. Now no matter where I go, I feel comfortable. I don't have to be hiding somewhere to take care of myself. I haven't gotten sick since I got the pump. I feel relaxed."

Candyann Charles says the same but adds another word: *hope.*

I ask Candyann, a diabetic since childhood, "On a scale from one to ten, how would you rate the insulin pump in terms of your quality of life?"

No hesitation. "A ten."

AFTER INTERVIEWING THE patients, I now understand the difference in the physicians' perceptions. The majority of physicians did not consider the insulin pump a new advance, because they simply looked at it from the end point, which is to give insulin and to get the numbers in line. From this point of view, the insulin pump is not dramatic. Only Dr. Agnes Gliwa had the empathy to understand that the insulin pump is a life-changing event for the patient. We have yet to find any number of cures, but physicians have made incredible strides in making the sick more comfortable. People like diabetics, cancer patients, and amputees are able to lead remarkably normal lives while waiting for a cure.

"Why don't more patients use the pump?" I ask Agnes.

"Because doctors have to be comfortable with the pump," she replies. "They have to learn about it and get used to it. They have to change the way they think and change what they are used to."

When pharmaceutical companies began direct-to-consumer advertising in the 1980s, many physicians objected. They asked, "How are patients qualified to judge?" Now I understand why patient empowerment and advertising are so important. You cannot count on your doctor to offer you what you need. Not because the doctor is a bad person or isn't trying to do a good job. It is just that the measure of success that your doctor has may not be the same as yours. The insulin pump and insulin injections both control glucose, but only one of the five endocrinologists to whom I spoke understood the effect on the patient's life.

The four endocrinologists who missed the point of the pump are more interested in what's being delivered than in the delivery system. They talk about an explosion of medications since 1994. More drugs have emerged in the last 15 years than in the last 1,500. The number of therapies is increasing with logarithmic velocity. The year 2000 saw a revolutionary breakthrough with the development of insulin glargine, sold under the brand name Lantus, which keeps the blood sugar constant. Lantus has the incredible advantage of rising to peak level instantly and then staying constant all day and night until it is time for the next shot. It means the patient doesn't pass out or get sick as the insulin and blood sugar levels bounce up and down all day long. It is a big deal to have a constant amount of insulin. With Lantus, a diabetic needs only one shot a day.

The years 2005 and 2006 were cataclysmic for applied physiology; that was when researchers developed drugs that release insulin from the pancreas. These drugs, called incretin mimetics after the hormone they imitate, also decrease the release of glucagon, a hormone that raises blood sugar. If you decrease the release of glucagon, blood sugar levels will not rise as much. If you want to feel smart, walk into your doctor's office and say, "Hey, Doc, I have been thinking about going on an incretin mimetic drug for my diabetes. What do you think?" You will feel very proud of yourself as you watch his eyes get wide. How do I know this will happen? Because of the 3,000 medical students and physicians I see in classes each year, only about 10 percent of them know about incretin-mimetic drugs. These are recent advances. If your physician or your loved one's physician is not a subspecialist in endocrinology, he or she may not know about them and certainly may have no idea how to use them. That is why, like Lorraine Brooks, today's patients need to be educated themselves and partner with their physicians.

CHAPTER 19

More Time for Loved Ones

The Revolution in Dialysis

M Y BOSS, DR. EDMUND BOURKE, chair of medicine at SUNY Downstate, has twinkly, happy eyes and a face prone to joy far in excess of the normal human being. In his early seventies, he maintains a level of energy in excess of most of our students. His curiosity and his hunger for wisdom and understanding are the qualities that define him. Each week, for as long as I have known him, he has taught in both morning report and in the special intern morning report in front of our freshest, most knowledgeable, and cutting-edge clique in the institution—and has managed to be ahead of them at every turn.

When the facts of the moment have faded from the memories of our students and interns, the greatest gift we instructors give them is our own enthusiasm to learn. Some might say that cutting-edge teaching would be better left in the hands of the more recently graduated; however, nothing better characterizes the goal of making our trainees lifelong learners than to have their chairman running faster than they are. No one would fault Dr. Bourke if, at his level of accomplishment, he were to retreat into the well-worn, comfortable shoes of physical examination teaching; the details of which have not changed for 50 years.

Besides being chairman, Dr. Bourke has also been a nephrologist for almost 40 years. I tell him that I will probably skip the discipline of nephrology, which has to do with kidney disease, as a topic for this book because I do not know of any major breakthrough in the field. But Dr. Bourke has a surprise for me.

"More than fifty years ago," he says, "life without kidneys became a viable option."

Before that time, having no kidneys meant suffering from uremia, the accumulation of waste products in the blood. It is as the patient were marinated in urine. Uremia makes people feel tired, confused, dizzy, light-headed, and generally lousy. When it is very severe, it causes coma and death. In 1943, Dr. Willem Kolff invented the first dialysis machine out of sausage casings and vacuum cleaners in Nazi-occupied Holland. Dialysis is the process of placing a very large catheter in the patient's bloodstream to move the blood in and out of the body so that it can be cleaned of waste. Dr. Kolff, who died in 2009 at the age of 97, spent the last years of his life on the faculty of SUNY Downstate.

Dr. Bourke continues: "During those days, dialysis was confined to those who were relatively young and did not have other serious illnesses."

As recently as the 1960s, there were so few dialysis machines that they had to be rationed the way we now ration organs available for transplantation. Only younger patients were chosen, so as not to "waste" a resource.

The chairman goes on: "We then began to be able to support those who were older or who had concomitant, comorbid conditions. The quality of life on dialysis became dependent on the amount of blood we could circulate through the artificial kidney. This is mainly due to the diseased vasculature of these patients."

The same diseases that lead to kidney failure—diabetes and high blood pressure—also damage the vascular system. Over time, the vessels become narrower and narrower. This narrowing of the vasculature makes it hard to get access to do dialysis. Twenty percent of the output of your heart goes through the kidney each minute. That is an enormous volume. In order to do dialysis, you must get a very wide access. A wide catheter must be placed to get the blood clean. Most of the physical problems of the procedure of dialysis stem from inadequate access and the infections that accompany it.

Dr. Bourke continues, "It is only in the last five years that nephrologists have taken on the breakthrough task of improving the circulation through dialysis vascular access."

If the vessels narrow, the nephrologist can reopen them. Technically, interventional radiologists could do the procedure, and traditionally they would. But they never see the patient again, so they don't know if the work is adequate for dialysis. Having the nephrologist establish the access means that the nephrologist can monitor the dialysis to see if the vasculature is adequately improved. The entire endeavor is called interventional nephrology.

Dr. Bourke explains, "This has resulted in faster blood flows into the artificial kidney. This leads to better clearance of the molecules of waste products causing uremia. This means that there is a better sense of well-being for these patients. This means the amount of time you have to be on dialysis with each session has been shortened. Try to imagine what it is like to have to only spend three hours on dialysis with each session, rather than five hours. The patient does not have to sit in a chair in a dialysis unit, but rather be at home enjoying the privilege of their grandchildren. Finally, by shortening the amount of time it takes to do dialysis, it opens up more space in each dialysis unit to accommodate more patients. Shorter hours per patient allows an economy of scale that was unimaginable in the past. The brand-new field of interventional nephrology allows all of this because of maintaining and creating high-flow, dependable vascular access. You can't clean the blood if you can't get the blood into the dialysis machine."

There is something about his saying "better sense of well-being" and "enjoying the privilege of their grandchildren" that makes me a little teary eyed, like I'm at a wedding. *Dearly beloved,* I think, *we are gathered here to witness the blessed union of the artificial kidney with the blood vessels of the patient in the holy bonds of dialysis. Separately, they do not achieve their sacred purpose, but joined together, they bring forth new life and a greater sense of well-being not possible for them separately.* Something beautiful and new is being created, and it's not just the whole new field of interventional nephrology. It is an evolutionary step in thought. Instead of a person who is a one-time consultant on a single procedure, the usual caregiver is taught the advanced procedure. The concept of holism takes a big leap up.

DR. MORO SALIFU is the newly minted chief of nephrology at Downstate, which has pride of place in the field. Not only was Willem Kolff, inventor of dialysis, on the faculty, but the first federally funded dialysis program in the country was started at Downstate. The first African American ever dialyzed was a Downstate patient. The portable "suitcase" dialysis machine was invented at Downstate by Salifu's immediate predecessor, Eli Friedman. Salifu himself is the first Ghanaian chief of the division. He is brimming with excitement, blazing a trail to a whole new way of thinking.

Salifu says: "Interventional nephrology has revolutionized the way we treat our patients on dialysis. It is a brand-new field."

"See?" Dr. Bourke, also present at the interview, chides me with a laugh. "I am not as 'over the hill' as you thought I was! Interventional nephrology is the only new subspecialty in internal medicine in the last twenty years."

Dr. Salifu tries to continue, but Dr. Bourke interrupts him, saying to me: "Everything else you are talking about is twentieth century; interventional nephrology is twenty-first century! Get with the program, Conrad, get with the program! Ha, ha, ha!"

When Dr. Salifu can finally get a word in, he tells me, with justified pride, "We are the first academic medical center in the country to have interventional nephrology in-house, in the hospital, that can do these procedures."

The timing was miraculous for one desperate patient.

Dr. Salifu explains: "One of the first patients had severe swelling of the neck and entire left upper extremity due to complete obstruction of the innominate vein [a very large vein near the collarbone that drains the head, neck, and arm]. This patient could not be dialyzed and roamed from place to place looking for help until she was referred to me." He adds empathetically, "She came to me crying. She was basically dying, really. But then I was able to reconstruct blood flow into the heart, relieving the venous pressure that was responsible for all the swelling. Now it is fixed. That is interventional nephrology."

Hope has a new synonym, and here I thought there was nothing new in nephrology.

EVERYONE KNOWS YOU can do a stent for a coronary artery in the heart, but few know about doing it for vascular access for dialysis.

"We can take blood vessels, like the subclavian artery, that have stenosed and open them," Dr. Salifu tells me. The subclavian (under the clavicle) artery is a main branch of the aorta and the source of the carotid arteries, which supply the brain. It also supplies blood to the arms.

Dr. Salifu adds, "We have patients whose vena cava [one of the veins carrying blood to or from the heart] has clogged off; we pass a wire into it and balloon it open."

Physicians are so specialized that many may not even know that vascular access can be restored. I did not know you could balloon open a subclavian artery. And a physician cannot refer a patient for a procedure he doesn't know exists.

"We can access the whole venous system," says Dr. Salifu. "The access points clot off. We can put in thrombolytics [clot busters] directly into the sites of obstruction."

Dr. Bourke pops in again: "Interventional radiology won't do these procedures as well. The nephrologist sees the effect on the patient because he is the long-term caregiver. The interventional radiologists don't see the patient coming in with their family who are upset that the patient is inadequately dialyzed. They don't talk to the family members who see their mother at home falling asleep in front of the TV nearly comatose. If you are the doctor taking care of the patient, you are connected with the result. Interventional radiology is not equipped to know what is going on."

If you are not watching results, looking immediately at effects, gathering data, and trying new things, you do not advance the specialty. In one sense, interventional nephrology is a closer monitoring of failure.

The nephrologist sees how a vascular procedure fails or is inadequate and is more likely to develop a new method of solving the problem, and hence advance new methods.

Dr. Salifu continues: "Interventional nephrologists have the right motives for doing their work. Interventional radiologists will not advance vascular access. They just do the procedure and get out. No research, no progress. The other specialties will not understand the clinical effect on the patient. They do the procedure and never know what happens next. We see the patient every day."

He gives me a case in point. To gain the vascular access required for dialysis, the nephrologist creates a hole in a patient's arm. It takes some time for the connection to become thick and strong enough to handle the input of a huge needle three times a week to do the dialysis. It takes about six weeks, and the doctor can feel the vein, which is normally thin, become thicker and more like an artery. The volume of flow becomes enormously greater.

In one case, however, the hole was not healing properly.

Dr. Salifu says: "I said, 'It has been there for four months.' It turns out there was a stenosis of the brachial artery. There wasn't enough flow into the fistula [hole], so it would never have matured. I took the patient into the lab and passed a wire. Now there is blood flow and the fistula matures. Another branch of medicine would never have understood this, and the patient would have been waiting around to this day for the fistula to mature."

He tells me about another instance, in which a patient had severe swelling of the neck and chest wall, with fluid accumulating in the chest around the heart and lungs, squeezing them off because of backflow from a clogged vena cava.

"I was able to reconstruct blood flow into the heart, relieving the venous pressure that was responsible for all the swelling and effusions," he explains.

THAT SAME NIGHT, I go with incoming nephrology fellow Melissa Rampal to meet the patient. Directly witnessing such dramatic new procedures and the birth of a new subspecialty is one of the most important things for Melissa's professional development.

"Interventional nephrology is the wave of the future," she says. "I just think no one knows about it yet. They don't know what we can do. This is the kind of thing I am going into nephrology for. I want to see what I can do to expand this ability to other hospitals that do not have it."

Melissa is a creative, open-minded professional. She is not going into nephrology just to be a dry cleaner for the human body. Melissa is going into nephrology to be on the cutting edge and to offer hope.

"It is really important for me to see the immediate effects of our work on people's lives," she says. "The patient does not understand how amazing the procedure done on him was. But I know. It's up to us to make sure people understand how much better what we have to offer is than in the past. We have to make them appreciate the breakthrough so they will have hope for the future."

I could not have said it better myself.

CHAPTER 20

Quality, Not Quantity

A Better Life for Cancer Patients

My boss, dr. edmund bourke (who, as I described in chapter 19, enlightened me about interventional nephrology), tells me one day that he is worried about one of our oncology fellows: "She is thinking she made the wrong choice and wants to drop out. She feels depressed and ineffective."

Knowing all about my optimism project, he asks me to speak with her. As an experiment, I set the oncology fellow the task of finding cancer patients who would have died or lived with excruciating pain just five or ten years ago without the treatments that we have today. For a few weeks, she searches and calls me each time she finds one. She listens to their stories of experience, strength, and hope. At the end of the process, she changes her mind.

"I'm going to stay in oncology," she says. "I see what I can do now. I just didn't understand before."

It takes a particular type of person to be a clinical oncologist, one who knows that she is a handmaiden to what, despite her efforts, may still be death. It is a deeply intimate specialty. Not everyone can take on this noble task. Dr. Jasotha Sanmugarajah and Dr. Gurinder Sidhu, two full-time clinical oncologists at SUNY Downstate, are among the breed. Satisfaction in being an oncologist requires altering your expectations.

Dr. Sidhu says: "Even though I know I am not always bringing cures, I know I am bringing help. I know that people are more comfortable because of what we do for them. They come weak and short of breath. We can control the disease enough so that they feel better."

Dr. Sanmugarajah says: "People come with certain goals that we can help them with. They want to live long enough to see their daughter graduate from college or to see the birth of a child. We can do at least that. We can control their nausea so they don't feel as bad. You have to readjust your expectations if you are an oncologist. We can't always cure, but I think we can always make people feel better. We can also make people feel that they are not alone."

Chemotherapy as an idea is terrifying to patients, who are not likely to know that over the last 15 years several entire new classes of antinausea medications have been developed.

"Ondansetron and granisetron are really amazing in their ability to make people more comfortable. Ondansetron was approved in 1991, and granisetron in 1993. They both inhibit the part of the brain that controls nausea. Aprepitant was approved in 2003 and also makes people much more comfortable," says Dr. Sidhu.

"Twenty years ago, all we had for nausea was compazine and metoclopramide. They were not strong medications, and they did not control the nausea and discomfort that comes with chemotherapy," says Dr. Sanmugarajah. "Even when we know we cannot cure the disease, we are still certain that we can make the time people have better time and more comfortable time."

Dr. Sanmugarajah—or Dr. San, as she is called by people who can't handle the musical quality of her Indian name—is the picture of calm clinical confidence and unflappability. She exudes a quiet intelligence and does not appear very emotional. The watchword of her existence is accuracy. People place their lives in her hands with regularity. People with cancer will live and die by the drugs and the doses she chooses. When you have such a serious illness, calm confidence is exactly what you want.

"I don't want to give people false hope," says Dr. San.

I won't be finding the exalted poetry of breathtaking advances here, I think.

But she continues: "Just because I don't want to give false hope does not mean there are not new drugs that work. Let us look at metastatic colon cancer."

Honestly, I would rather not look at metastatic colon cancer, because she is going to review the statistics, and I will have to change the title of this book from *Routine Miracles* to *Occasional Improvements*. Dr. San smiles the quiet-intelligence smile again.

"In 1990," she says, "all we had was 5-fluorouracil for colon cancer. In 1995 we get irinotecan, then in 1998 to 2000 we get oxaliplatin and bevacizumab (Avastin). The survival starts to go up. The new drugs take the survival, even for metastatic cancer, from six months to nine months to twelve months and now to thirty-six months. So the new drugs have added a lot of survival for colon cancer."

Must be true. After all, Dr. San is the high priestess of the temple of No False Hope.

"Remember," she says, "there are genetic mutations developing in all of us every day, but we don't all develop cancer. That is because the immune system detects these mutations and gets rid of them before they become cancer. People develop cancer because those mutated cells are not killed and they start multiplying. This is why a deficiency of immunity can predispose to cancer." She adds, like a stake in my heart, "Few cancers can be cured."

"Then what keeps you going?" I ask her and Dr. Sidhu. "Don't you get frustrated just sitting around watching people die?"

"Sure you get frustrated," Dr. Sidhu says. "You change your goals. I had a woman in the Kings County clinic with metastatic breast cancer who was about to die. I put her on Taxol and Herceptin, and she got enormously better. In four weeks she was a new woman. Okay, she didn't get cured, she may not live forever, but this is enough gratification for me to have something to feel good about what I am doing. These drugs work. We can't cure everyone, but as long as we are extending their survival and making their symptoms go away, that is good enough for me."

Dr. Sidhu and Dr. San are clear that they cannot cure very much, but they can make people feel better. They can relieve symptoms and, even if the patient does not live longer, they are both 100 percent sure they can make him or her live better.

"Targeted therapy is going to decrease the amount of chemotherapy we use in the future. The fear of chemotherapy is going to decrease," says Dr. San.

Targeted therapy is a drug that inhibits a specific enzyme, gene, or protein of a cancer cell and leaves the rest of the tissue alone. Chemotherapy cannot tell the difference between good and bad cells very well. It kills any fast-growing cell. Targeted therapy is like a missile that blows up only the target and not the innocent people next door. There is no collateral damage. So, in the final analysis, Dr. San has something better than no false hope: real hope.

DR. BILL SOLOMON is the perfect clinician-scientist. A man in his mid-fifties, graying and balding, he spends one part of each day with patients and the other part managing National Institutes of Health (NIH) grants. His perspective is deep. He stands halfway between the molecular world of the lab and the emotional world of the patient responding to chemotherapy. I join him at the end of a meeting with his research team.

"Let's look at the 1950s, when people first discovered that breast cancer needed estrogen to grow," he says. "Fifty years ago, we would have to remove the ovaries of a woman to stop the production of estrogen. We did the same with men and prostate cancer in removing the testicles to stop testosterone. The exciting thing now is that the pace of discovery is much more rapid. We have thousands of people working in these endeavors to understand these pathways. We have over thirty drugs that are targeted therapy for various forms of cancer."

Tamoxifen as an inhibitor of estrogen is relatively old. It was in use thirty years ago, even when I was in medical school. The idea is fantastic: a medication that will block the effect of estrogen on breast cancer without the need for removing the ovaries. Tamoxifen decreases the recurrence of disease and clearly lowers mortality. Over the last 10 to 12 years, drugs have also been developed to inhibit aromatase, the enzyme that produces estrogen. Anastrozole was approved in 1995, and letrozole was approved in 1997. Aromatase is present not only in the ovary but also in adipose, or fat, tissue as well. Aromatase inhibitors prevent the growth of breast cancer. They prevent the recurrence of breast cancer after a mastectomy. Anastrazole and letrozole prevent death by stopping breast cancer cells that don't get cleaned up by chemotherapy. And the patient gets to keep her ovaries.

A woman feels a lump. She gets a mammography. She gets a biopsy. Estrogen and progesterone receptors are checked on the biopsy. If they are positive, she gets an estrogen receptor antagonist such as tamoxifen or an aromatase inhibitor. But she may need to have a surgical procedure to see if the cancer has spread into the lymph nodes in her armpit, known as the axilla. Women with breast cancer have typically all had to have their axilla dissected. If a woman has cancer in the lymph nodes, she must get extra chemotherapy and get radiation to the axilla. There is currently no test to tell whether the cancer has spread into the axillary lymph nodes without removing those nodes. Big nodes don't necessarily have cancer; small nodes are not necessarily free of cancer. This is a big deal for the quality of life of these women. Besides the discomfort and complications of any surgical procedure, removing lymph nodes in the axilla blocks the lymphatic drainage of the arm, which can lead to swelling of the arm. Permanently. The swollen arm often leads to infections of the arm, which can recur for the rest of the person's life. For nearly a century, that is what many women with breast cancer had to look forward to.

In the 1990s, the sentinel lymph node biopsy procedure was developed. This is truly a reason to be cheerful. In the operating room, dye or radioactive contrast material is placed in the first, or sentinel, node. The doctor removes that first node to see if there is cancer in it. Cancer spreads sequentially from the breast to the sentinel node, then to subsequent nodes. If the sentinel node has no cancer, the other nodes will be free of cancer 99 percent of the time. If the sentinel node is clean, the doctor does not have to dissect the rest of the nodes. No swelling, no infections.

Unfortunately, operative methods are some of the slowest practices to change in medicine. Although proven nearly 15 years ago, it has taken most of that time to make this more elegant biopsy the standard of care. Close to 220,000 women a year are diagnosed with breast cancer; close to 220,000 will be spared chronic and recurrent arm infections, making the sentinel lymph node biopsy procedure one of the greatest advances in oncology.

BESIDES BEING A full-time clinical oncologist, Dr. Sidhu is also a teacher at the medical school. After several discussions, this tall, elegant, stately, intelligent man has climbed on board my optimism train. I wonder if he is faking it just to keep me happy.

"No, I really feel it," he says. "I really think we can do things for people that make them feel better."

In the time of the great 19th-century physician William Osler, even the attempt to treat cancer was considered the sign of a charlatan or quack. Dr. Sidhu has me speak to one of his patients, Ms. Violet Burgess. Ms. Burgess is a quiet, polite 56-year-old woman who has breast cancer. After years of being disease free, Ms. Burgess has recently learned that her cancer has recurred.

"I don't really feel anything," she says. "It is not like the chemotherapy I had that could make me feel sick or lose my hair. I get the Herceptin, and it goes in, but I don't feel it."

Herceptin (a brand name for the drug trastuzumab) is a targeted therapy; that is, it targets specific receptors on the surface of breast cancer cells and leaves the normal cells completely alone. It is an antibody against one antigen on the surface of the breast cancer cell. It turns out that another victory of basic science is the discovery that 20 to 30 percent of breast cancers express the human estrogen receptor type 2 (HER-2) in increased amounts. It is not, therefore, a universally effective drug for everybody with breast cancer. But it does give a painless extra punch for one in three patients. It can add a couple of years to people's lives. The risk of relapse can decrease by 50 percent.

Herceptin is one of Dr. Sidhu's reasons for optimism: "We have trastuzumab, which controls disease with very little cost. By *cost* here, I mean there is very little discomfort for the patient. Monoclonal [single-antigen] antibodies may not be as hugely potent as chemotherapy, but they don't make you sick."

Liver cancer is another area to see a significant advance in targeted therapy. Sorafenib is a drug that inhibits angiogenesis, or the formation of new blood vessels that feed the cancer. During trials, the data monitoring board considered the effect of sorafenib to be so dramatic that the members decided it would be unethical to continue a placebo-controlled branch of the study. Overall, sorafenib can add a couple of months to the life of a patient with liver cancer. I know what you are thinking: "big deal, a couple of months." But look at it this way: sorafenib is oral—you can stay home or go on a cruise ship when taking it; the patient suffers few adverse effects, since sorafenib is targeted to the cancer; and a few extra months of healthy life is better than an infinite amount of death. Since President Richard Nixon declared war on cancer in 1971, there have been more than 100 trials of medications to stop liver cancer. None of them worked. Now we have an angiogenesis inhibitor that at least does something.

Interventional radiology is also being brought to bear in the fight against liver cancer. It is the most extraordinary of extraordinary new branches of medicine. Using probes, needles, and wires, an interventional radiologist is able to enter parts of the human body that previously would have been accessible only by surgery. The doctor can completely avoid the side effects of surgery and can do biopsies and offer therapies never dreamed of in the past.

DR. ERICK LANG is an interventional radiologist who chaired the department of radiology at Louisiana State University (LSU) for 35 years. He ended up in New York by way of Hurricane Katrina, which practically wiped out LSU.

When I meet him, Dr. Lang is placing a special probe into the liver of a patient with a huge cancer mass.

In an Austrian accent that makes him sound like Arnold Schwarzenegger, he explains: "This man has a liver cancer that will kill him before he is able to get a liver transplant. The probe I am putting in will deliver radiofrequency energy that will decrease the burden of the tumor so that it might be small enough so he will live long enough to get transplanted. High-frequency electrical currents are passed through the electrode, creating heat that destroys the abnormal cells. Between you and me, I do not think it will work, but the patient wants to try. It just keeps the tumor burden down so he can stay on the transplant list."

Dr. Lang is in the interventional suite today working with people from the manufacturer of a new machine that will deliver energy into the tumor so that it will shrink. He is learning a new method with new technology that is safer and less damaging to the surrounding tissue.

I ask how long he has been doing this sort of thing.

"I have been doing interventional radiology for forty-six years," he replies. "I did the first angiogram of the coronary arteries in the world in 1959. Radiofrequency ablation [RFA] is the latest thing. We have tried liquid nitrogen to freeze the tumor [cryoablation], embolization of the artery feeding the tumor, and alcohol ablation, but none of them have been very effective."

Although Dr. Lang has his doubts about the benefits of today's procedure for this particular patient, with his history he is able to see each individual procedure as a step in the march of progress. The next step in experimentation for treating liver cancer would be to have Dr. Lang insert a radiofrequency ablation probe to "cook" the lesion, while at the same time trying to shrink it with sorafenib. That study has not been done yet. I explain to Dr. Lang my idea that contemplation of our accomplishments energizes us more to seek the next breakthrough. I figure that with 46 years in his specialty and his status as a chair of a university program, he will have the long view.

"I completely agree with this approach," he says.

AN INCOMING CHIEF resident, Brandon Smaglo, is at the opposite end of his medical career. He has known since he was a medical student that he wanted to be an oncologist. He will enter into a fellowship in oncology the year after his chief year. Brandon is one of those heroic figures who knowingly takes upon himself the enormous task of treating cancer patients. He has a calling. There are many medical students of extraordinary intelligence. There are many residents who are capable of working hard. There are many physicians with large hearts who are strong enough to bear the responsibility of life-and-death decisions. But only a handful combine these attributes of intelligence, hard work, and responsibility with a willingness to care for the dying.

Brandon is already mentally prepared to be an oncologist. He has different expectations. He is not living only for a cure. His goal is to give his patients a better life, if not necessarily a longer one.

He says: "Even though the targeted therapy may not always extend survival, the time you do have is much better. We may not be able to extend the length of the life, but we can enhance the quality of the life. I would argue that if you are going to be treated for a cancer and you are going to get some kind of standard, nonspecific chemotherapy, you may live for three years, but it is going to be a crappy three years, and you have to go in and out of the hospital. You may be incapacitated. If you use these pills as directed therapy, you may live the same amount of time, but you are able to live your life as you would normally and productively for most of the same time, then we are doing a better job."

Brandon is wise for his years. We doctors quickly forget how horrible things were when there were no treatments at all. Many of us regret that we have no cure rather than appreciate what we are able to do. By considering the quality of life that we are able to provide, we can gather solace and strength as we search for a cure. Of the scores of doctors I interviewed, those who appreciate what they *can* do are the most satisfied and productive.

"I mean, everybody is going to die at some point," Brandon says. "As physicians, if we can't enhance the length of someone's life but can enhance the quality of it, then we are doing a pretty good job. That's what I think a lot of these medications are doing. They are keeping people out of the hospital: you can take the therapy on your own and you are not having the complications of therapy. This is what I think was knocking people down for so long with these things. You are in and out of the hospital not because of the disease but with some of the complications of the treatment of the disease. These treatments that we have now, they may not necessarily make you live much longer, but you are able to live better."

CHAPTER 21

Stealth Victories in Oncology

Nothing quite captures the terror of illness like a diagnosis of cancer.

I ask oncology resident Brandon Smaglo (whom I introduced in chapter 20) to approach cancer patients as potential interviewees.

He says, "Of the four cancer patents that I spoke with, three of them did not realize they had chemotherapy, and two did not even know they had cancer . . . which I found very interesting."

Interesting? I think. I know I'm a dramatic guy, but even Brandon has got to admit that this is astounding.

Brandon says: "I have two people with multiple myeloma, and when I referred to their disease as cancer, they were shocked, and said 'What!? You mean I have cancer now?!' I told them, 'You have had cancer for years, and that is what you are being treated for.' And they were blown away by this. They then said, 'Oh no, I am going to have to take chemotherapy!" and got very upset. I said "No, you are *on* chemotherapy: that's what these pills are that you have been taking.' And they had no idea they were being treated for cancer."

Multiple myeloma is a type of cancer of the plasma cells in bone marrow. Plasma cells are white blood cells that make antibodies. In myeloma, cancerous plasma cells make excess antibodies, or immunoglobulins. These immunoglobulins have no clear function, but they are made in such large amounts that production of normal immunoglobulins ceases. They act like a paranoid schizophrenic who throws out his refrigerator and television to make room for spy detection equipment. Normal function ceases. The cancerous plasma cells then destroy the bones to the point where they become so brittle that just a cough will fracture a rib. The abnormal immunoglobulins clog off the kidneys till the patient ends up on dialysis. The overgrowth of plasma cells chokes off the production of normal blood cells and causes anemia. When infection enters the body, the plasma cells stay stuck on their overproduction of useless immunoglobulins instead of making an antibody to control the infection. The victim dies of infection. The body makes colossal amounts of immunoglobulins, but not against anything useful.

Two of Brandon's patients have no idea that this is what their doctors are fighting or how they are fighting it. He says, "They did not know the thalidomide they were on was chemotherapy for myeloma."

Thalidomide is a story of triumph and tragedy. It is like the Zen Buddhist story of the farmer whose horse runs away and all his neighbors say, "How terrible—what bad luck." The farmer says, "Maybe." The next day the horse returns with ten wild horses. The neighbors exclaim, "How wonderful! What good luck." The farmer says, "Maybe." The next day, the farmer's son falls and breaks his leg while working with the new wild horses. The neighbors say, "What a tragedy! How sad!" The farmer says, "Maybe." The next day the army comes through the town conscripting all the young men into the army to fight a war. Because of his broken leg, they leave the farmer's son alone. All the neighbors say: "How lucky!" The farmer only responds: "Maybe."

In the 1950s, thalidomide was approved in Europe as a drug for morning sickness in pregnancy. Everyone says: "How wonderful!! What good luck!" An administrator for the U.S. Food and Drug Administration, Frances Kelsey, says "Maybe," and refuses to approve the drug because of inadequate safety studies. Everyone says, "What a tragedy! The drug is not available here. What bad luck!" The following year it becomes clear that thalidomide causes birth defects, and the drug is instantly banned. It is not found anywhere in the United States. The Americans say: "How wonderful! No birth defects develop here!" Two years later in Israel, a patient is suffering from a terrible form of leprosy. The pain is so bad the patient cannot sleep. "What a tragedy! How unlucky."

"Maybe."

Dr. Jacob Sheskin is the physician in the small Israeli hospital. He is desperate to find something to help his patient sleep through the discomfort of his leprosy lesions. He finds a bottle of thalidomide on the shelf in his hospital. He remembers that thalidomide has sedative effects. It would not have been found on the shelf in an American hospital. "What good luck!"

"Maybe."

Dr. Sheskin gives two tablets to the patient. Not only does the patient sleep through the night, but a short time later all the leprosy lesions resolve! After a clinical trial, thalidomide is proven to be an excellent treatment for resistant leprosy, and, in a few years, all the leprosy hospitals are closed. "What good luck!"

There was only a single tenured professor in the United States doing research on thalidomide. This professor, at the Rockefeller University, determines that thalidomide inhibits a substance known as tumor necrosis factor in patients with myeloma and gives them the same benefits as intravenous nonspecific cytotoxic chemotherapy *without many of the side effects.* In 2006, the FDA grants approval to thalidomide for myeloma therapy.

What good luck . . . maybe.

BRANDON GOES ON: "The patients did not know they had cancer, and did not know they were on chemotherapy for myeloma. We also had a patient with chronic myelogenous leukemia who did not know he had cancer. He was on Gleevec [imatinib]."

Gleevec is oncology's miracle of miracles. It controls the disease in a whopping 95 percent of cases.

"He was not coming to his appointments. Gleevec costs thousands and thousands of dollars, and he was not taking the pills and even lost them. He came saying, 'I need more.' He was an undocumented immigrant, and we had to go through leaps and bounds to get them for him and do a lot of under-the-table things with the drug company to get him his pills. He had no idea what he was getting. He had no idea he was getting a miracle in a pill. He did not understand that you could not just go down to the corner drugstore and pick up some more."

We are living in a world where doctors have to jump through hoops just to do their jobs.

Brandon points out, "The best treatments that we have to offer are still on patent, they are very hard to get, they are very expensive to get. One of the things we do very well here is get people medications by working with the system, which is very impressive. A lot of times patients don't realize that just having the medications is a miracle for them. Obviously they *should* get the medication; that is what we are here to do, we are here to help."

We demand ethical physicians, but some practitioners have to go so far as to lie in order to save lives. The managed care problem is forcing them to be unethical in order to be compassionate. There are physicians who will put their licenses, careers, and jobs on the line to get uninsured patients the care they need.

Brandon continues: "If these patients are uninsured or undocumented immigrants, and if you look at it from a purely bureaucratic standpoint, they don't deserve the medication. They are not insured, or they are not part of our country. They are not paying taxes into the system. Should they get the medication? Sure they should. They have a disease."

Brandon may not realize it, but he is implementing the word of the father of modern medicine, Sir William Osler, who advised medical students, "Get denationalized early. The true student is a citizen of the world, the allegiance of whose soul, at any rate, is too precious to be restricted to a single country. The great minds, the great works transcend all limitations of time, of language, and of race, and the scholar can never feel initiated into the company of the elect until he can approach all of life's problems from the cosmopolitan standpoint."

Still, despite the lofty ideal, Brandon has to think about the hard facts of the matter.

"It's what we are here to do," he says, "but I don't think the uninsured or undocumented immigrants realize they are basically getting a 'donation' of thousands and thousands of dollars in treatment from the government or from a drug company. It is a lot more money than some of these people would see in their lifetime. They would never be able to scrape together the money they need to get these treatments on their own. It's just interesting to me that they do not even realize a lot of times what they are getting and how they got it. And it is not just any medication, but they are getting these new therapies which allow them to avoid a horrible alternative such as old treatments."

"SO TWO OUT of the four people I talked to did not know they had cancer. Three out of the four did not know they were on chemotherapy. It's incredible."

He says: "This is where oncology is at; this is why it is really cool right now. We are getting to a point where people are afraid of diseases, but they don't even realize they have the disease they are afraid of."

"What?! Can you say that again?"

"You say the word *cancer* to somebody, and it has such a horrible stigma to them. They are afraid of cancer, but they don't realize they have the disease that they are afraid of. They don't realize that they have cancer, which is what would inspire terror in them. You put the person out of peril, and unfortunately they don't understand what is going on with them. For standard chemotherapy, you have to do a lot of monitoring and do a lot of other tests. Now they take a medication with very few side effects, so they come in for a prescription and a few blood tests and away they go, so they don't even realize what they have, and what they are taking."

Well, doesn't this summarize the title of this book nicely? "Routine Miracles" are now so common that cancer patients don't even know they have cancer.

The biggest stealth victory in oncology is not in treatment at all but in prevention. Smoke-free environments are routine now. The No Smoking light on an airplane is always lit. In many cases, the legislation that bans smoking is based on protecting employees from exposure to tobacco smoke, not on abridging the rights of smokers to kill themselves with their own smoking. But, as a side benefit, smoking control has led to more than a 25 percent decrease in lung cancer over the last 20 years. Direct deaths from tobacco are at about 450,000 a year in the United States—300,000 from emphysema and 150,000 from lung cancer. By comparison, cervical cancer kills fewer than 4,000 people a year, colon cancer, 50,000 a year; and prostate cancer, 28,000 a year. Adult smoking rates have started to fall below 20 percent for the first time in a century. Taxes on cigarettes have helped bring the number of smokers down. By restraining people from lighting up in public, we have saved 37,500 lives from lung cancer.

Prevention methods in other areas have also saved hundreds of thousands of lives: the mammogram, the Pap smear, and the colonoscopy. All three of these methods are extremely effective in detecting early disease that doctors can actually do something about. As much as 95 percent of colon cancer deaths could be prevented if colon cancer screening methods were universally applied.

Gardasil is a vaccine against the human papillomavirus (HPV) and can prevent as much as 70 percent of cervical cancer. Significant battles won, all below the radar for the masses of people who will now never have suffered from cancer.

The most common cause of cancer death in the world is liver

cancer, which can arise from chronic hepatitis B and C infections. Chronic hepatitis C is the most common reason for needing a liver transplantation in the United States. There are not enough organs to go around, and a large number of people die while on the transplant list. For those fortunate to receive a transplant, the medication tacrolimus, discovered in 1994, prevents rejection of the liver by inhibiting the lymphocytes that would reject it.

Gastroenterology fellow and routine-miracle fan Naveen Anand delivers to me this exchange from an interview he's done with the grateful girlfriend of a chronic hepatitis patient: "We were so happy when he got the transplant because he got so much better, but now we know that his liver had cancer in it, but we did not know until after they took the liver out. The hepatitis made it so I was more like his caretaker rather than his girlfriend or his wife. Now he is all better, and he has come back to me. He is so happy that he got this gift. He is not tired all the time, he can work, his mind is better."

Naveen asks, "So you didn't even know that hepatitis can give you cancer?"

"It can?" says the shocked girlfriend.

"Yes," says Naveen, "the chronic inflammation of the liver from the infection causes cancer. The medications like lamivudine, entecavir, and adefovir prevent the inflammation and cancer."

These one-pill-a-day medications are also essentially completely devoid of side effects.

AND THEN OF course there are the cancers that we can't prevent but can control in an overwhelming percentage of cases, such as myeloma and acute promyelocytic leukemia. Acute promyelocytic leukemia has jumped from being the worst form of acute leukemia to being the most curable.

"She was almost dead, she was bleeding to death," Dr. Bill Solomon (see chapter 20) says when describing the acute leukemia of patient Pauline Gordon.

Acute promyelocytic leukemia comes with a cascade of clotting that consumes all the blood's clotting factors and platelets. You start to bleed from every orifice. In the general patient with acute leukemia, there are 6 to 12 weeks between diagnosis and death. With class M3 acute promyelocytic leukemia, it is even worse. A patient can come in essentially bleeding to death, like Ms. Gordon.

"Promyelocytic leukemia is a form of leukemia that is so bad that you have to treat it the same day or the patient dies," Dr. Solomon says. "Pauline Gordon got daunorubicin and ATRA."

ATRA stands for all-trans retinoic acid; it is a vitamin A derivative. The cancer cells that cause leukemia want to stay immature forever and simply reproduce. ATRA compels the cells to differentiate and grow up. It acts sort of like a parent who kicks a 25-year-old adolescent out of the house, saying "Get a job!"

Dr. Solomon says, "She was hours away from dying, she was bleeding to death."

"So you are sure the ATRA snatched her away from the jaws of death?" I ask Dr. Solomon.

"No question," he replies. "Absolutely ATRA drags you back from death and has very few side effects . . . ATRA compels the cells to differentiate. Patients don't bleed to death anymore."

He finishes with the superzinger: "Promyelocytic leukemia has been the worst form of acute leukemia. Now it is the only really curable form. About ninety percent of patients treated with ATRA and chemotherapy get cured—totally cured—without bone marrow transplantation."

There is something about the way he repeats the word *cured* that gives me a warm, fuzzy feeling.

I follow up with Pauline Gordon, who is the 39-year-old mother of two children, ages 8 and 11.

"I was bleeding in my mouth and gums and I had red blotches in the skin of my arms. I was given my diagnosis right away," Ms. Gordon says.

She feels quite well. She had no idea how bad the disease is that she had, despite the fact that she was, she says, in shock, nervous that she was going to die. She vividly recalls being in the intensive care unit (ICU) for bleeding. I am surprised that she has heard of ATRA and knows her medications. Since her original diagnosis, she has been in remission and is on maintenance chemotherapy. For Ms. Gordon, the treatment is just a collection of pills and injections she gets. Since leaving the ICU, she's had no fear. All she knows is that she takes pills and comes to the hospital for injections every few months. It really is all very routine for her. The questions I usually ask about family support, feeling a burden on others, feeling resentful, the impact on her spirituality, and the emotional impact are not greeted with any depth of feeling. All she remembers is feeling too tired to take care of her children. I presume that her lack of enthusiasm comes simply from the fact that she was well treated and the serious problems quickly resolved. Acute leukemia for Ms. Gordon is a matter of scheduling and inconvenience at work, not that she was almost dead.

She *is* grateful. But, overall, her feelings are rather subdued, even when she says she knows that treatment is much better than in the past.

"Yes, it is a miracle I am doing so well given the serious nature of having leukemia," she says.

DOCTORS ACCIDENTALLY DISCOVERED the promyelocytic leukemia of another patient, Ms. Moore, on a complete blood count done for another reason.

"I got chemotherapy, and I am on ATRA now," she says.

That's about it. She doesn't report any huge emotional or spiritual impact. Her brush with death is straightforward and routine.

"The only thing that is frightening is the bone marrow biopsy," she says. "The only emotional impact on me was from having to stay away from my kids while getting chemotherapy."

When I ask how her treatment compares with past treatments, she just doesn't know. Ms Moore is glad she is doing well and feels very satisfied with her caregivers. Does she know that until only recently she would likely have rapidly bled to death? Nope.

I have a mixed response to these two patients, especially Ms. Moore. On the one hand, they should not know anything more than that their disease is controlled and that they are free to live their lives without fear. On the other hand, part of me wants to shake them up and to frighten them about what would have happened to them in the past without ATRA. Of course, I don't. How it *was* is history. People, especially those who never witnessed firsthand the lack of treatments, are not going to remember. It's just part of the condition of being human: we forget.

PART 6

Patient Empowerment
Empowers Us All

CHAPTER 22

Accentuate the Positive

HIV Patients Still Struggle for a Normal Life

IN 1991, WHEN I was still at St. Clare's Hospital, I got a call from Lincoln Hospital in the South Bronx. This was pre–Rudolph Giuliani New York. Badlands. Gangsters. Gangbangers and violence.

The operator said, "We have a call to Dr. Fischer about your brother being in the emergency room."

My brother is a drug dealer, so I was not completely surprised when they told me over the phone, "Your brother has been shot."

I went to the Bronx. As I walked in, he saw me.

"Brother-man! Bro! How you doin'?"

The physician looked bored and busy. He was standing over my brother, removing bullet fragments from his chest and neck with a forceps.

He immediately said, "You're the brother who is a doctor? Good. Can you finish this? I have to go."

He nodded toward the glove box and handed me the forceps. It was an interesting and, in a way, comical scene. A self-service hospital that had so many gunshots coming in that the doctor wasn't needed to tend to a shotgun wound to the chest and neck as long as the blood pressure was good.

"What happened, Jerry?" I asked my brother.

"Well, you see, bro, I was up here getting something, and, well, I was in this empty lot and, well . . . someone tried to rip me off, so I popped him in the face. I left, but he had a lot of friends. Then all of a sudden, every house seems like someone is running out with a bat or a stick. I thought I got away; they were all chasing me, when I bumped up against one of his friends with the shotgun. And, well, you know . . ."

I wondered how much of this was true. You could never be sure, and I wondered if it mattered. I just knew it wasn't as bad as the .38-caliber bullet he'd taken in the leg a few years before that had shortened the leg by two inches. There was no point in talking, except for amusement.

My brother Jerry is a few dozen points of IQ above genius. He graduated from one of the best prep schools in New York. My mother thought it would be safe there. Jerry, however, always said, "That's where I learned to get all the really good drugs, with the rich kids."

He talked, I listened. *He really is a charming guy,* I thought as I (the one with only average intelligence) pulled the bullet fragments out of his neck. *A generous, well-meaning guy. Really.* Like the time he insisted on driving up to college to collect me and all my stuff. He did show up to get me. In a stolen car. I was arrested and released. He went to jail for having some cocaine on him, and I later went to bail him out. I was 18.

"Listen, Jerry," I said after I'd finished extracting the bullets. "I will go to meetings with you. I will take you to Narcotics Anonymous. Let's go. What are you doing with yourself? Where are you going?"

"Well, bro, I never really wanted to be anything else except a dead playboy. I had three apartments, two cars, a different girl in each. Now that I am finished up as a dealer, I really don't have any other goals."

INCREDIBLY, MY BROTHER lucked into a marriage with the kind of woman who can turn a man's life around. They worked together and were friends, and he married her to help her get a green card. My sister-in-law is a young Israeli who is a straight-and-narrow type of person. After she got the green card, she and Jerry fell in love. My brother had had lifelong substance abuse problems despite his off-the-scale IQ. However, he loved his wife very much, and with the super-stable woman in his life who despised his drug-using friends, he was, after getting married, the cleanest and most functional of his life. Besides that, he was a mushy, romantic kind of guy, and although he did not love himself enough to stay clean, he did clean up much more to make her happy. All very romantic. Just like out of a movie.

I HAD JUST recently completed my fellowship when I got a call from my sister-in-law. She had a cold, she said, or maybe bronchitis, or maybe a little pneumonia. She was coughing and short of breath when walking up stairs. Huh?

"Short of breath?"

"Yes," she says. "I can't make it up a flight of stairs without stopping."

"Does anything come up when you cough?"

"No, but I do have some white stuff in the back of my throat that scrapes off when I touch it."

I know what this is, but it doesn't make any sense. I tell her: "You need to go to the hospital. Now!"

In the hospital emergency department in 1994, a dry cough, short-ness of breath, and thrush (fungus) in the back of the throat was a snap diagnosis. My sister-in-law had pneumocystis carinii pneumonia (PCP) and candida in her throat. She had contracted AIDS.

My brother was stunned. He turned out to be HIV-negative. Appar-ently a boyfriend, of which there had been very, very few, had transmit-ted it to her before she married Jerry. My brother was disappointed to learn that he was negative.

"If she dies, then I am going to also," Jerry told me. "I should be the one to have it, not her. It doesn't make sense, and it is not fair."

Despite a lifetime of irresponsible behavior, my brother never for a second even considered leaving. Actually, quite the opposite—his life was tied to hers.

She recovered briefly, then received the only AIDS medications available in 1994, which did not yet include protease inhibitors. She was stable for a few weeks and then developed lactic acidosis and hepatic steatosis, a very, very rare complication of HIV medications. It was so rare that, at the time, there were only a handful of case reports, and the doctors at Cornell Medical Center went so far as to do a liver biopsy. My sister-in-law fell into a coma and died. At her express wish, her family was never told that she was HIV-positive; they were told she died of cancer, and they took her back to Israel to bury her.

My brother lost all reason to be clean. At the age of 40 he took up using drugs with a needle and set out on a not very subtle attempt to ruin his life. He drifted to Florida, where he was arrested several times for minor traffic violations. Like driving the wrong way down a one-way street, clearly high. He told the police officers his name was . . . Conrad Fischer!

I was summoned to appear in court in Florida. Jerry was completely directionless. Disappointed he was not HIV-positive. When he got arrested then, it was worse than ever before. My brother developed terminal drug addiction. A few months later he was dead from an infection of his heart after shooting drugs that destroyed the valves. My brother died of a broken heart.

OUR MOTHER'S LIFE has always been her family. Her main goal was to have six children and then manage grandchildren. She only made it to three children before she got divorced. Never able to accept drug addiction as a disease, my mother still sees it as an environmental failure.

"If your brother had been supported enough," she once told me, "this would never have happened. I cried every day for years over my dead son."

To this day, my mother has never recovered. My sister-in-law was a very sweet lady who kept her son clean and was the closest thing she'd ever had to a daughter among her own three sons and four grandsons.

When one person is ill, it is never one person who is affected. It is the whole group of people around that person. When my sister-in-law died, a few months short of living long enough for protease inhibitors to snatch her life from the jaws of death, my brother died with her. And part of my mother died with them.

Nine months after my sister-in-law's death, combination antiretrovirals with protease inhibitors came out. Had she had her diagnosis in 1995 instead of 1994, she would have lived. I have never told my mother this. It would only make her losses worse. The wait for antiretrovirals killed my sister-in-law, precipitated my brother's relapse, and broke my mother's spirit.

Neither patients nor physicians can overestimate the need for medical research to move fast.

LI IS A 42-YEAR-OLD mother of two children who was fortunate to have found out her HIV status in 1996, when it had just become clear that combination antiretroviral therapy was highly effective. In a flash, the situation changed from certain death to managed disease. Li's trouble began when she started to feel short of breath. At first her doctors told her she had asthma and treated her with inhalers, which didn't work. Over several months, she progressed to the point of being in a coma, losing 50 pounds, and being placed in an intensive care unit for pneumonia. Her doctors finally performed an HIV test; it was positive. Her husband was unable to understand or accept it. He was HIV-negative, and the transmission was from a past boyfriend whom Li suspects knew his status but never told her.

In the opposite situation from my sister-in-law, Li kept her life but lost her husband.

"I weighed a hundred pounds and could not get out of bed for months," she says. "I was weak and fragile and could not take care of myself. My rent went unpaid and the bills were piling up. He left me just when I needed him the most."

Li made a slow recovery. With combination antiretroviral therapy, she got better and now is somewhat overweight and much happier.

"I lost a lot of friends at the time who could not accept it," she says. "My parents found out, and they were my main support, but . . . they thought I was going to die at any moment. I believe in family. I was pregnant with my son, and all I thought about was having a healthy baby."

Li was severely anemic at the time I met her during her first pregnancy. Because of this, she could not take AZT, the original medication that prevents the mother-to-child transmission of HIV but has the unfortunate side effect of causing anemia. She also would not take a blood transfusion because of her own personal beliefs.

"I am not a Jehovah's Witness," she says. "I just don't believe in taking transfusions."

Because of other HIV medications and good luck, her child today is healthy and beautiful.

"I believe in family. The most frightening thing for me was thinking I would not be there for my children. I feel fortunate, and blessed, very blessed, to have two healthy children while being HIV-positive."

Li's HIV, although resistant to multiple medications, is sufficiently controlled to allow her to lead a normal life, at least physically.

"I thank God for the medications," she says. "If you are HIV-positive and they ask you to volunteer for research on new medications, you should do it."

When I ask her if she feels fortunate, Li says, "There is always someone worse off than you. Cancer will eat you up alive in no time. I had a cousin who got bitten by a mosquito and died of dengue a few weeks later and left three small children with no mother."

However, Li has lived with a man for the last six years who does not know her HIV status. She had a second child who is also healthy, but she is not fully happy.

"If this is the extent of my happiness, I am okay with it," she admits.

She just cannot bear to bring herself to tell her partner about her HIV status. She is diligent about practicing safe sex, and she knows he is HIV-negative.

"You become more sheltered when you are HIV-positive. You have to be careful who you tell," she says.

We have talked many times about her disclosing her status to her partner. I have gone so far as to offer to invent a story in which both of them test at the same time and I pretend to find out just now that she is positive, like it just happened, so that her partner will not become angry at her. Li just cannot bear to do it.

"I know he will leave me," she says. "You have to hear how they talk about people with HIV. I say, 'You don't know what it is like for people. You have to put yourself in their shoes,' but it doesn't work. I know he will leave me."

JUST LIKE INTERVIEWEES with other diseases, Li is happy to share her story, but only using a nickname known to a few family members who know her status. Despite advances in treatment, the social stigma of HIV is still considerable.

One of my interviewees is so anxious that she is worried even to have her initials used. "Please don't even use my initials. I am scared someone will know I'm HIV positive." Anonymous is a 48-year-old woman who found out in 1989 that she was HIV-positive when she went to donate blood for her sick child. Anonymous is the only person I interviewed for this book who would not allow me to use her name or even her initials. I choose to call her Anonymous rather than make up a false name. *Anonymous* as a word reminds us of how isolating having HIV can be and how far our society still has to go in terms of accepting people with this illness.

"When my son was sick," Anonymous says, "he needed surgery on an aneurysm. I was stunned to find I was positive. I wasn't promiscuous. I wasn't a drug user. My husband was HIV-negative. The only thing I can think of was a blood transfusion I had received several years before. All I thought about was *Please, God, let me live long enough to take care of my son*. I did not realize what this meant for myself until later. I never expected to live this long. My son turned twenty-one this month."

"How were you told?" I ask.

"They called up over the phone and told me. All I remember was they told me never to have any more kids."

HIV has a tremendous effect on families.

Anonymous says, "My husband became consumed with my being HIV-positive. All he did was research to try to find a way to help me. He was driving me crazy, really. Finally, I had to leave him. I felt I was holding him back. I felt he should be with someone who was healthy. He couldn't understand. He is still my best friend. To this day, he still calls me up and says, 'You know what I just heard about such and such new treatment.' I know HIV had a lot to do with us breaking up."

When I ask what she is grateful for, she first mentions the medications that keep her alive. She then adds that she is grateful that HIV has taught her tolerance. Apparently, the tolerance that Anonymous feels for others is not reciprocated by what she feels from others. Hence, she feels compelled to completely hide her identity. Nowadays she has a new and great relationship with a man she met in an online dating service for HIV-positive people. Within that community, at least, she feels comfortable to be herself.

BILLY FIELDS, 57, is an HIV-positive, completely-out-in-the-open gay man. He has found strength, not stigma, in the community, and gave me permission to use his full name. He has been HIV-positive for 16 years, and I have been his doctor for 14 years so far. He can tell me to the exact day that he found out he was HIV-positive because it was the same day his father died. Throughout our talk, however, is the clear feeling that Billy knows how lucky he is.

"When I came to see you, I had four T cells," Billy says.

T helper cells are the main cell that is infected and destroyed by HIV. The normal value is above 600 to 700. So when Billy says he had 4 T cells, he's indicating that he was only weeks to months from death.

"The first time that I did not think I was going to die," he says, "was when I met you. I woke up every day prior to that thinking I was going to die."

Billy has a new type of faith in his caregiver. Although he implicitly trusts me, he always does enormous homework.

"You have to educate yourself," he says. "You can't go into the doctor and just say 'I am sick'; you have to look into things."

Billy says to fellow patients: "Educate yourself! In this type of environment, you have to work harder than your doctor. You have more time than they do, so go to the library or the Internet and find out about things. Then be selective in who you choose as a doctor. Make sure it is someone you can talk to and stick with him. But make sure you come into the visit with information." On the one hand, Billy has tremendous faith in me personally not to let him down; on the other hand, he never just sits back and lets me tell him what to do. Billy does not see it as contradictory. Patient empowerment is something that really developed with HIV and has become more widespread. Your doctor is now, in a way, your consultant in your own investigations and choices. Some doctors feel that if patients become more knowledgeable and independent, the doctor-patient bond will weaken. But Billy shows us that patients who are independent minded and well educated can help foster a sense of kinship with their physicians. Partnership with an educated patient encourages the growth of the human relationship that is the heart of our profession.

"What is the most frightening thing to you, Billy?" I ask.

He responds, "When I get sick and I do not know what will happen. I also feel like I let you down when I get sick."

I never heard something like this before. It confirms to me the strength of our bond.

I ask Billy if he lost any relationships when he was diagnosed as HIV-positive.

"Oh no!" he replies. "My family is very supportive. And if you were going to lose friends, then it is better to find out right away, because they weren't really your friend to begin with. My mother always told us, 'When someone gets sick, come calling,' so in my family and with my friends, I only got closer to people. I have tremendous friends who go way out of their way to help me. And I go take care of other people when they get sick."

When I ask him what gives him the motivation to go on, I am stunned and amused by the response.

"I love to play tennis! I want to stay alive to play tennis!" He adds: "You have to be involved, to do something to make sure funding is there. You have to play your part. It is kind of like a child saying, 'What did you do in the war, Daddy?' You have to do something. That is why I sit on committees and go to the capital to lobby for money for treatment."

ONE DAY IN 2008 I went into the waiting area, and as I scanned the room, I saw someone atypical: a well-dressed, attractive woman with blue eyes, blonde hair, and a stylish scarf. I assumed she was an administrator, or more likely a drug company representative.

I called out for my next patient: "Victoria Poole?"

The stylish woman stood up.

Victoria Poole is my age, 44. She is an educated, extremely well-traveled heterosexual white woman with no risk factors for HIV. She has known that she is HIV-positive since 1992, when, while living in San Francisco, she had the fever, fatigue, and rash we now know is associated with acute HIV infection.

"They did not know what I had. I did not fit. But, seeing as I was a single woman in San Francisco and not knowing what else to do, they tested me for HIV."

Like Li and Anonymous, Victoria would never have found out her status if testing was done only according to risk factors such as Billy's. You cannot tell who is HIV-positive simply by looking.

Victoria says, "They gave me my diagnosis over the phone. They were not used to seeing many women with HIV. They didn't know what to do with me, but they told me I would most likely be dead within five years. There wasn't much available in terms of medications at that time, and my T cells were still high, so I was not on therapy. I did not know what to do, so I went to a support group. I hated it. It seemed like a lot of people sitting around complaining and feeling sorry for themselves.

"I decided to take a different route and became, for lack of a better word, an activist. I figured if I was going to die soon, I wanted to make sure that my life had some meaning. Overnight I developed 'AIDS star syndrome.' I went to the White House, met Bill Clinton. I now work in the HIV in the Workplace program worldwide. I know that I had to do something. I knew that I was atypical. As an educated white woman, I knew I had more access to have my voice heard than others, so I had to fight back. This is what gave my life purpose and, at that time, at least, gave me energy. I am grateful that there are medications, even though I have not had to use them. I have been in seventy-eight countries. But now I just want to be normal."

AIDS IS A SPECIAL CASE in the area of diseases for which we can offer quality of life, though not a cure. Everyone can and should take hope from the fact that Li, Anonymous, Billy, and Victoria are alive and well. Their stories illustrate more poignantly than any other patients' the importance of the physician's role not only as healer of the body but as guardian of the spirit. HIV patients are the original advocates of patient empowerment, which many physicians fear weakens the doctor-patient bond. Yet throughout the country, HIV patients like Li are sharing with their doctors the difficulties and dreams that they cannot tell their own husbands, boyfriends, and partners.

Victoria is extremely clear: "The hardest part about HIV for me is not the fear of death. It is getting into a relationship. I still feel like a pariah when it comes to this. I have had a lot of bad reactions from men. They get angry, they threaten to hit me. They are just not very educated about the subject. Sometimes I feel I want to write *The Straight Man's Guide to Safe Sex.*"

Drug development is great. And Victoria is grateful for a lot of things, but the social stigma of HIV and the profound loneliness that can come with it are still heartbreaking. She feels simultaneously the pain of isolation, as well as the good fortune of access to care.

"It is not like I am a woman in rural Malawi," she says. "I know if I get sick, there are options."

She leaves me, her doctor, with her fondest wish: "I just want to lead a normal life. At this point I would just be happy to have a boyfriend, sing in a band, and do some pottery."

CHAPTER 23

Dermatology Treatment as Antidepressant Medicine

Doctors and Patients Working Together

A MANDA DOYLE JUST finished her first year of medical school a few weeks ago. She has already seen doctors do many miraculous things. But her sense of wonder at new therapies is not as sharp as the bad smell some negative faculty creep has sprayed on her: Eau de "Being a Doctor Was So Much Better before You Were Born."

Older physicians have poisoned Amanda's mind with the narrow-minded idea that practicing medicine just isn't satisfying anymore because, Amanda tells me, "We used to have more autonomy. We have a lot of family friends who are doctors, and I just heard this when I was volunteering in the hospital when I was in high school."

This is not the first time that I have heard this argument, and I am profoundly deflated to hear this argument coming from such a young student barely having begun medical school. What drives older physicians to volunteer this sort of "information" to new students? Why the impulse to dampen their enthusiasm? I worry that I am too late to save Amanda from this epidemic of narrow mindedness.

Amanda has been doing research on the effects of skin diseases on patients' psychological states.

"People would just start crying even when they took the survey," she says. "I thought I was just handing them a piece of paper with a few questions on it, but they would spend half an hour talking about how miserable they were. I was studying acne, and people would talk about how devastated they were that their boyfriends didn't want them around their families. It was just very . . ." Her voice trails off.

As a second-year student, not yet numb to the pain that surrounds a physician, Amanda sometimes has difficulty translating the suffering she sees into words.

"It was just very profound," she continues. "They would wear turtle-necks even in the summer. They would wear cover-up makeup even to bed . . . Some people would just avoid leaving their houses entirely because they did not want to meet anyone."

AMANDA DIRECTS ME to Maria, a patient suffering from psoriasis, which comes from antibodies that attack the skin. Patches of silvery scales develop. They can be as small as a fingertip or cover the patient from head to toe. Psoriasis is a common condition affecting 2.2 percent of the population, or more than 5 million people. We don't know what causes it. We do know that 60 percent of people with psoriasis report it to be a very large problem in their lives. Besides the obvious discomfort of itching, people with psoriasis are also uncomfortable about how they look.

Maria tells me, "People who didn't know what it was would wiggle away from me. They were hesitant to hand me a paper or touch anything on my desk because of it" She says, "[People] didn't want to speak to me. They thought it was contagious. They thought that if a little flake fell on them, it would spread to them.

"My own mother wouldn't let my nieces and nephews hug me. She wouldn't let them touch any of my clothing, because she thought the psoriasis would spread to them. We are not on speaking terms right now because of this.

"If I lay down on a bed and the kids would sit on the bed, my mother would get all upset and start yelling for them to get up and wash themselves. She wanted to keep everything of mine separate from everyone else, things like my cups . . . I felt isolated and frustrated and angry. I felt that other people did not want me around because of it.

"My mother is very religious, and she thought I brought it upon myself by not taking care of myself. My mother thought the psoriasis got worse because I did not want to pray about it."

AMANDA CLEARLY UNDERSTANDS the heartbreak of Maria and other dermatology patients.

"One woman told me that she could not bear to be near mirrors," Amanda says. "She just avoided ever looking in a mirror."

I ask Amanda to accompany me on an interview with Dr. Alan Shalita, chairman of my hospital's dermatology department.

Dr. Shalita graduated from medical school the year I was born. I usually see him as a gruff man.

"We have a camp in the summer for children with skin diseases," he tells us. "They can go to the camp and feel normal and accepted, because everyone has a skin problem. There are enormous psychological issues with the diseases we treat. It is a whole specialty that we have here of psychodermatology."

I am delighted to hear of such a wonderful idea.

Dr. Shalita's clinical nurse specialist, Carol Duncanson, joins us. Carol is in charge of ultraviolet light treatments, which selectively uses the segment of ultraviolet light that is therapeutic without the part that causes a suntan or skin cancer. When someone has to undergo ultraviolet light treatment, it means he or she has a serious, life-altering skin disease.

Carol says, "I should have a psychiatrist's couch in my room. All of our patients have stories to tell about how their psoriasis is affecting their lives. There is virtually no patient who doesn't have an enormous psychological impact of the disease. You can walk around with cancer and nobody will know. You can walk around with kidney disease and nobody will know. You walk around with skin diseases and everybody knows. It messes with your self-esteem. I had a young man who was not doing well in school. He was suspended on a regular basis, and he was acting out at home with his mother. He had psoriasis on eighty-five to ninety percent of his body. His mother was very concerned about putting him in camp, because with shorts, the kids would see lesions, and he would be ostracized."

Dr. Shalita interrupts. "But we have a camp for kids like this."

Carol presses on. "No, I mean normal camp. He was started on etanercept, improved within a few weeks, and has been ninety percent clear ever since. There have also been times that we have taken him off, and he has periods when his disease will stay clear for a few months."

Etanercept is a biological agent approved in 1998. Biological agents are antibodies produced in a laboratory to mimic a part of a natural biological molecule. They are incredibly specific. The difference between steroids and biological agents is like the difference between a bomber and a sniper: steroids inhibit the growth and activity of anything they touch, whereas biological agents can be tailor-made to remove a single molecule out of the system. Etanercept removes the molecule known as tumor necrosis factor (TNF).

Carol continues, "Let me say something. I have young people who don't date or who lose a relationship due to psoriasis. They become introverts, and it's very difficult for them. Etanercept really brings them back to life."

For many people, dermatology has connotations of superficiality, yet it covers diseases that have some of the most psychologically destructive impacts of all the medical diseases. You might think heart disease or cancer, the biggest killers, would draw the best students in medicine, but dermatology is actually the single most competitive of the specialties to get into. Effective therapy transforms the patient's life. After interviewing Amanda, Maria, and others, I have to take back the nasty things I've said about trying to get the best students unlocked from chasing dermatology. They are working to rescue patients from an emotional death, if not a physical one.

DURING MY INTERVIEW with Maria, she tells me about her own transformation: "I started to have psoriasis when I was twenty-one, and now I am 35. It started as a patch on my lower back, and the Lotrisone wasn't working as much. They switched me to vitamin D cream, Dovonex, but the psoriasis was getting worse and the cream was irritating. It went away, then came back all over my body. New creams would work for a while, but not much. Ultraviolet light didn't work after two months, and neither did vitamin A cream. Then pus started coming out, including on my face. Only methotrexate made a difference, but we were concerned about toxicity.

"The Enbrel [the brand name for etanercept] was really dramatic. Ninety to one hundred percent of the psoriasis cleared up for me after years of having this problem. It cleared up first during the summer. Now I was able to go out without covering myself up. I am more confident. I don't have to hide myself. All the negative feelings I had before have been changed into positives. This new drug was like taking two antidepressants.

"It was like being brought up out of the ashes; it was like Lazarus being resurrected. And it was not just me being healed, it was like my whole family was healed."

After her success with Enbrel, Maria moved to a different state. Her new doctor wanted to put her back on methotrexate. She switched doctors to get the therapy she needed.

Her advice to other patients: "Keep on plugging. Eventually people will just adapt to you instead of you adapting to them."

WHEN THE INTERVIEW with Maria is over, I ask Amanda again why she has the impression that medicine was better in the past.

"Patients are more responsive and smarter," she replies. "It kind of puts the doctor in a different position. Traditionally, you would just go to the doctors and listen to whatever they said. People would follow us like it was a religion."

I say, "Well, in this case, if the patient had listened to her new doctor, she would—"

Amanda interrupts to finish the sentence herself: "Be in a world of trouble."

Ah! We finally achieve some mutual understanding. Maybe one day Amanda will come around to my way of thinking after all.

CHAPTER 24

"Listen to Your Patients"

Treating Pancreatic Disorders

"**I** AM DR. FRANK GRESS'S poster child!" says his patient Erin Grove as her voice comes bubbling up through the phone. "How is my friend doing?"

I am always taken aback when patients ask about the health and happiness of the doctor. Like a lion who'd had a splinter removed from her paw, Erin is brimming with gratitude even though it has been years since she was in the care of Dr. Gress, chief of the Division of Gastroenterology and Hepatology at SUNY Downstate.

"I had horrible, uncontrollable, unmanageable pain that did not respond to medications," Erin says. "All I had was side effects of the medications. I had the pain for four and a half years before I met him. I went from hospital to hospital across the country. I couldn't even get a diagnosis. I was dismissed as a crazy woman. They sent me to two different therapists. I would sit in therapy making them laugh. That was hilarious. One would repeat everything I said. I was paying him, and I was making him laugh. I was vomiting outside and was in terrible pain, and he said to my husband, 'How do you feel about this?' We were at a family conference. My husband said, 'How do you *think* I feel about this? I am fucking happy!' So we got up and left. The next therapist said, 'How do you feel?' and I said, 'I feel like shit.' He said, 'Oh, we are not doing well?' Then he said, 'We are going to visualize the pain.' I said, 'I don't want to fucking feel it! Why would I want to *look* at it?' And we left."

"Did they put you on psychiatric medications?" I ask.

"Yes, they put me on a tricyclic antidepressant, amitriptyline, which was wonderful for a twenty-eight-hour nap."

"How many doctors did you see for your pancreas problem before you saw Frank?"

"About forty."

"You saw forty doctors?" I say, my voice squeaking up to a high pitch.

Now I know why they tried shunting Erin—with chronic pain, multiple normal scans of the abdomen and pancreas, and her irreverent pain-in-the-ass personality—off to psychiatry. Burned-out caregivers often believe patients exaggerate their symptoms in order to gain something.

ILEA KHAN IS a fourth-year medical student and a petite young lady whose appearance often leads patients to ask, "Are you sure you are old enough to be a doctor, honey?" or "Nurse, can you find my doctor?" Ilea lets it roll off her.

"That's just because I have better style than the faculty," she says with a wink.

Ilea can wax poetic for a half hour straight about the things her faculty know and teach her. Her favorite word is *fabulous*. There is one thing, however, that Ilea does not find fabulous. It is the quick assumption that patients exaggerate illnesses in order to gain something. Her "amazing," "wonderful," and "fabulous" faculty have no idea that they are polluting the soul of an enthusiastic physician-to-be by inculcating in her the idea that people exaggerate illness to manipulate the caregiver. In the emotional-endurance obstacle course of being a caregiver, it is very difficult to remain present and receptive to the suffering of others. In the face of so much suffering, it is a defense mechanism, blame the victim.

ERIN GROVE FELL right into this trap.

"I went to Johns Hopkins," Erin says. "I went to the Cleveland Clinic, I went to everyone you could think of in Manhattan. It was a who's who of GI specialists in the United States. I even got in to see David Skinner, who was the president of New York Hospital. All my CT scans were normal. My blood tests, the amylase and lipase, were also normal. Then I got a new test called the trypsinogen activation peptide, which was abnormal, and that was how the diagnosis was made. I got sent to the pain clinic at Cleveland Clinic, and they thought I was nuts. I went back to New York, and they were out of ideas. I was deteriorating, and no one had an effective treatment for me. I kept going in and out of the hospital. Finally they said, 'We have a new doctor coming in. He does all sorts of weird things with scopes.' They asked me if I wanted to try, and I said, 'Oh yeah!'"

Dr. Frank Gress has been said to look like Clark Kent on his way to change in a phone booth. Besides being the chief gastroenterologist, Frank is perhaps the world's leading authority in the procedure known as the endoscopic ultrasound (EUS), in which a sonogram machine attached to the tip of a scope allows the physician to see what was previously completely undiscovered except through open abdominal surgery.

Frank explains, "A gastroenterologist went from being simply a specialist with a lot of knowledge about disease making intelligent comments but not being able to actually do anything much, to a practitioner in a cutting-edge, state-of-the-art, technology-driven field. The sonogram, or ultrasound, that used to be placed on the abdomen for a fuzzy, indistinct image can now be placed into the center of the body on a fiber-optic scope."

Frank is the author of the only textbook on the endoscopic ultrasound, yet even in his own city, patients would not know to go to him for help.

You cannot seek out a doctor for a test you have never heard of.

Endoscopic ultrasound, the greatest triumph of recent gastro-enterology, is routinely available, as long as you know it exists and where to find it.

In addition to being a master of EUS, Dr. Gress practically single-handedly invented the best method to date of stopping the excruciating abdominal pain that arises from chronic pancreatitis. He figured out how to inject medication into the main trunk of nerves that cause the pain, a procedure called a celiac block, by using an EUS to locate the celiac plexus of nerves, which is between the stomach and the spine. Prior to EUS, it was possible to try to medicate the celiac plexus of nerves with CT scan guidance, but it wasn't as accurate. While the patient is inside the CT machine, the doctor advances a needle through the body, through the organs and tissue around the target, and then rescans and tries to put the needle right on the plexus. It is like build-ing a ship in a bottle.

Erin Grove was one of the first patients whose pain was controlled by celiac block.

"Frank saw me in a hospital in Long Island," Erin says. "He did the EUS and started to do celiac blocks on me. The first one did not solve it. But I kept going back and got more injections into the celiac trunk. The pain went away! And now I haven't had pain for three years."

"How did your disease affect your relationships?" I ask.

"It certainly tested my marriage. I was married for only two years when I got the pain. My husband is still looking for a rabbi to see if there is a lemon clause in the Jewish marriage contract.

"The biggest problem was people not believing me when I kept telling them there was a problem. They kept accusing me of being an alcoholic. When I got the diagnosis, they finally believed me. The most frightening thing was a loss of control. The pain made it so I could not make rational decisions. I was not able to live my life the way I wanted to. The celiac block made it so I could have some normal basic function. The pain made me feel I was a burden on my husband."

"The worst aspect of your experience was just the pain, right?" I think this is an obvious question, so I'm not prepared for Erin's answer.

"Oh my God, no! It was the financial aspect. We almost lost our home. I wasn't able to work. I had to sell my jewelry so I could buy medications in Canada. My mother gave me her engagement ring to sell, but I couldn't do that. We had to fly and stay in hotels when we went to all these hospitals, and insurance doesn't cover that. I met Frank when the pain was so bad that I collapsed on the street. The ambulance brought me to the nearest hospital. Frank was at the hospital they brought me to."

"What has had the greatest emotional impact on you?" I ask.

"The feeling of helplessness," Erin replies. "You feel helpless. There is nothing you can do. You just lie there."

"What did you learn that is most helpful?"

"Don't give up," she says. "Speak up. Open your mouth. I don't care that these people had medical degrees. I did not think what they were saying was right. Don't take no for an answer."

"Do you think having a lot of knowledge about your condition gave you more trust or less trust in the doctor?" I ask.

Erin is clear: "You have to educate yourself. There is a lot of information available electronically. Being more knowledgeable does not damage your sense of faith or trust in the doctor. You still have to have trust. It's just that there are a lot of knuckleheads out there with medical degrees."

"What helped you get through having all this pain the most?" I ask. She replies, "Humor!"

"How do you think your treatment compares with what was done in the past?"

"It is miraculous."

Her choice of the word is unsolicited.

"I don't think I could have done anything differently," she continues, "because what I had done did not exist before. I am grateful for all these advancements. I am grateful for these developments. I am grateful for these improvements. I am grateful for science. I believe in science."

But Erin begs the doctors in the audience: "Listen! Listen to your patients."

LUVIA BERNARD'S STORY is eerily similar to Erin Grove's. She has pancreatitis, but no one knew it for a long time. Despite sonogram after sonogram, CT scans, and blood tests, Ms. Bernard still had no diagnosis. She had upper abdominal pain just below the end of her sternum. Pancreatitis pain can be incapacitating. It ruins lives.

"They told me to stop drinking, but I told them I did not drink," Ms. Bernard says. "Nothing helped. The pain was so bad, I was depressed all the time, crying all the time, sad all the time. I thought about killing myself. They did not know what was going on with me. The doctors sent me to a psychiatrist. For two years they couldn't find anything. They just told me it was in my head, because the tests were all normal. I couldn't do anything. I couldn't work. I couldn't pay my bills.

"I was so scared. There was so much frightening to me. I thought I had cancer and nobody wanted to tell me. My boyfriend left me because I was in pain all the time and I couldn't do anything."

Ms. Bernard eventually came into the care of Dr. Frank Gress and underwent an EUS.

She is one of the lucky ones. Even in the technology-driven world of modern medicine, endoscopic ultrasound is a procedure done by only a small percentage of gastroenterologists. Despite years of pain, she found the man who could save her.

In a few minutes, Dr. Gress determined by an endoscopic ultrasound that Ms. Bernard had chronic pancreatitis. It had never been diagnosed because the tests that she'd had could not detect it. Although the pain did not go away overnight, in an instant her depression dissolved into relief.

You cannot overestimate the power of a simple diagnosis. Although the cause of her pancreatitis remained obscure, just knowing the cause of the pain changed Ms. Bernard's life and that of her family instantly.

"My family was so depressed with me," she says. "All they could do was stand around and watch me cry. It was so difficult for my mother because she could not help me. My daughter was so depressed about what she saw going on with me, she started having to take antidepressants. She should have been in college having a good time, but she saw me crying all the time. It had a very bad effect on her."

Even though her medical therapy has not begun at the time of our interview, the relief in her voice is overwhelming.

"I thank God that I now know what I have," she says. "I can get my life back. It's not all in my head. My family is so grateful."

Ms. Bernard's tone is devoid of resentment. Another type of person might be brimming with anger and resentment over two years of misdiagnosis and the failure to refer her for the EUS. She believes that people try to do the best they can with what they have and know.

She says, "I pray for the doctors to have more knowledge, more equipment, and more tests."

To my hearing, it is touching that she simply prays for doctors to have more equipment and more tests. She doesn't know how precisely right and accurate she is.

She advises other patients, "Don't ever give up hope. Keep going."

T.C., A RETIRED FILMMAKER and fellow pancreatitis sufferer, says essentially the same thing: "Keep trying! You have got to search for the solution."

T.C. has had chronic pancreatitis for more than ten years.

"Sometimes the pain is very sharp, sometimes it is stabbing, sometimes it goes down my leg." T.C. runs short of words to describe it. "The celiac block procedure I had from Dr. Gress eased the pain to a dull roar, and sometimes it made it hardly noticeable. Pancreatic enzyme pills helped, but not much. Oxycodone helped. The benefit of the block was dramatic and started immediately. So far, it is doing its job, and the pain has decreased a lot.

"The celiac block made me a nicer person. I wasn't as crabby, I wasn't as sharp with people. Sometimes the pain is very paralyzing. The most frightening thing is thinking that it would get worse and worse."

"What is most hopeful about your experience?" I ask him.

"To know that there is a way out; I just have to find it," he replies. "You have got to search for it. What is most depressing is thinking nothing could be done. It is very depressing when you think there are no options. Pain makes it so you can't concentrate on anything else.

"I kept trying till I found someone who could do something about this. In the past, I didn't find anyone who knew anything about it or who knew what they were doing. Nothing existed twenty years ago for this, I know that. I am in pain, but I feel lucky about this: I feel hopeful that there is help, and this is what relieves my depression. I feel lucky to have found someone who knew what they were talking about."

T.C.'s life was a horrible mass of suffering. It wasn't much of a life at all. In an endoscopic procedure that takes less than 30 minutes, his life is changed. Now think of all the people not in Dr. Frank Gress's reach—maybe yourself or a loved one someday. We need more Frank Gresses. But the epidemic of negativity spread by medical school faculty isn't helping their numbers to grow. Older faculty look back wistfully to their days of autonomy. But for Erin Grove, Luvia Bernard, and T.C. to regard their physicians as all-knowing instead of human beings would not have served them or the profession.

"NO ONE COULD figure out what I had," says Deborah La Pointe. "I didn't drink. I was doubled up in pain. They thought it was my gallbladder. I had my gallbladder taken out, and I woke up in pain. I was thirty-four years old and healthy. I had constant abdominal pain. They told me I had a hiatal hernia, which I didn't have. They told me I had reflux disease, which I didn't have.

"I was very diligent in finding out what was going wrong with me. I didn't just sit around. I got a stent put into the duct by another doctor, but it didn't make any difference. The pain was horrible, it was phenomenal, I couldn't function. I couldn't even take a walk. It is really incapacitating. The pain takes over your whole body. It is a constant, gnawing pain. Eating was not an option. My family and my husband felt helpless because there was nothing they could do for me. It made me much more isolated. I didn't see people, I couldn't go out. The most frightening thing was not knowing what I had. I thought it might be cancer. I had my gallbladder taken out for no reason.

"Then one doctor said he knew a very good pancreatic doctor . . ."

Dr. Gress did an EUS and found that Ms. La Pointe had pancreas divisum, a failure of the pancreas to grow into a single gland.

"For me the celiac block was a godsend," Ms. La Pointe says. "Each block would last about five or six months, but even if it would have only lasted three months, it was a huge difference for me. The celiac block changed my whole quality of life. I know this did not exist in the past. Even now, the other doctors did not know how to do this procedure. There were chat rooms on the Internet about pancreatitis, and everyone knew not to go to a gastroenterologist who did not specialize in the pancreas."

"What message would you want to give to doctors about your experience?" I ask.

There is a pause.

"You really want to know?" she asks with a laugh. "Be more open minded. Be open to other diagnoses. The doctors need to be more thorough, and they need to say, 'Okay, what else could this be?' When a treatment is not working, they need to see if there is another issue going on. A lot of doctors get fixed on their own specialty and what they have been trained to do. They don't go beyond the box they are in, and that is the problem I was finding. When the treatments were failing, they would think it was still just a problem in their own area.

"I have been fortunate to be able to give other patients insight into what their disease is. Doctors are not God; I know that. They do what they can do. Patients have to go on the Internet and help themselves. You have to exhaust everything. If what they are giving you is not working, you can't just take that . . . You have to put yourself in your own hands a little bit. It took me nearly ten years to get this figured out."

Ms. La Pointe's attitude surprises me. I would have been brimming with resentment at being shuttled from doctor to doctor for ten years before stumbling on what I had. But Ms. La Pointe is rational, practical, and forgiving. In the 21st century, there is no expectation of the doctor being all-knowing. If there is, both doctor and patient need to recheck their premises and try again. This is a forgiving, compassionate stance. Doctors and patient can search together for the diagnosis and treatment.

Perhaps our older physicians miss the unquestioned "priestly" qualities of the past. The faith-healing quality of ordering the demon of disease to be exorcised from the patient.

Now we are less mythological and archetypal in visage, but a heck of a lot more useful.

Perhaps the physician is now a guide to take you and him together to the shores of known understanding and ability, and then help each other, go farther.

CHAPTER 25

Gratitude in the Attitude

Informed Cancer Patients Trust Docs More

B RIDGET TULLOCH IS a 58-year-old cancer patient who is taken care of by oncologist Bill Solomon at SUNY Downstate. Ms. Tulloch originally came in with a dangerously high white-cell count and was diagnosed with chronic myelogenous leukemia (CML). Researchers have determined that CML is caused by a chromosomal abnormality that produces tyrosine kinase, the enzyme that, in turn, produces the disease. Control or eliminate the abnormal tyrosine kinase, and you eliminate the disease. The discovery of this translocation as the cause of CML is a triumph of modern science. Here at least is one cancer that we know the definite cause of.

Bill describes the effects of the disease when he first encountered it: "The first patient I had with CML was a twenty-year-old marine who was in incredible shape when he entered the marines. He found he couldn't do the huge marches in training at Parris Island. He went to the infirmary and found he had a white cell count of 1.5 million, with the normal being less than 10,000. At that time, all we had to offer him was the alkylating agent busulfan. All busulfan could do was lower your white count. This was purely cosmetic treatment. You lower the white count but cannot change the ultimate outcome, and he was dead within two years."

That was 20 years ago. Things are different today, says Bill: "We took a disease that essentially killed almost everybody and was incurable and now can control almost everybody." He explains, "In the 1980s we were experimenting with bone marrow transplants if you had an identical twin. Even if you had an identical twin, the mortality from a bone marrow transplant was 25 percent. Ten years later, we developed alpha interferon, which is a naturally occurring substance in the body. This was the first drug therapy that had any real effect, but even though the cell counts got better, only a very, very small percentage got cured—only about 2 or 3 percent. It took another ten years to develop imatinib [Gleevec], which is an inhibitor of tyrosine kinase. Now as many as ninety-five percent of patients can be treated with Gleevec, and their chromosomal abnormality . . . goes away. It also meant you did not have to take a chance on that risky bone marrow transplant, which had such a high mortality."

Bill calls Gleevec "the home run of this century's advances in oncology."

Bridget Tulloch is on Gleevec. There is a little complexity. She is a Guyanese immigrant without the insurance to cover the cost of the medication. Gleevec costs $5,000 a month. Through a program called Compassionate Use, Bill Solomon has worked with the drug company Novartis to get Ms. Tulloch her medication for free.

Bill introduces me to Ms. Tulloch, who is very enthusiastic about her doctor.

"Dr. Solomon has gone above and beyond the call of duty of an exceptionally high service to help me," she says.

She has brought him a token of gratitude, a fountain pen, and is trying to press it into his hand. Her expression of gratitude makes Bill so uncomfortable that he virtually flies out of the room. It's easy to feel unappreciated in medicine, and her gratitude is the octane of the soul.

"I know that there are many people who died but who, if they had Gleevec ten years ago, would be alive," Ms. Tulloch says.

I am surprised that she is so well informed. Her sense of history and appreciation is rare. Many people saved from life-threatening illnesses question little and simply take the prescription to the pharmacy, fill it, and take the pill. This book would be a success if only that single treatment registered on you as a "Routine Miracle."

"How do you know this?" I ask, delighted to have found one lady who understands both the gravity of her illness and the blessings she has received.

Her answer: "Because I read."

Many doctors pooh-pooh the idea of patient empowerment out of fear that patients will not respect them if they become partners in care. In fact, patients have more respect and gratitude for doctors who hear them out.

"So you know that ten years ago you would have had to have a bone marrow transplant?" I ask Ms. Tulloch.

"Yes, I know . . . There are miracles. Somebody has to bless you for this. I am so fortunate, and I am a sinner. Even when I am watching television and I see what a surgeon or a specialist has done for somebody, I bless that person because he has been given a gift to cure people, and many people don't come back to say thank you. Dr. Solomon is a special person. If I'd had to have done it for myself, I wouldn't be here today. We have to start being grateful spiritually, emotionally, and financially for the things that are happening for us. We cannot divorce ourselves from spiritualism and from knowing that there is someone higher that is working through people like Dr. Solomon and like you to write this book."

Wow. Ms. Tulloch had no idea she would meet me today. No advance warning. No time to prepare such an accurate statement of my mission.

Ms. Tulloch has been on Gleevec for three years.

"I have to work through this challenge," she says. "I am so blessed, I can't be negative. When I fall down, I get up again. The social worker has worked to have my bill reduced, and Dr. Solomon has given his approval to do all this for less. Are you going to tell me this is not a miracle? Why should I not try to be kind to people or to pass on this kindness and this miracle to someone else? When I call the company to make a delivery, I always say to the people at Novartis, 'For those who forgot to say thank you today, I thank you on behalf of all the other patients whose lives you have saved. Thank you.' You have to say thank you, it's so important.

"I am no Goody Two-shoes, believe me. I have been saved. I say, 'Thank you, God, for the opportunity to be here.' If I didn't have this disease, I would be taking everything for granted."

I simply sit next to her and listen, not wanting to interrupt the slightest molecule of the homily being constructed in front of me in central Brooklyn.

"I don't have the money," she says, "but I have the love. Once, I admitted to Dr. Solomon that I did not take my medication because I forgot it. He came to hug me so firmly, I cried. I cried because here was somebody wanting to help me, and I missed my medication. Since then I have never missed a dose. "

"What has been the most frightening thing to you?" I ask.

"Nothing" is her firm response.

"Why has there been nothing frightening? You have cancer."

Ms. Tulloch continues to nearly knock me out of my chair with her statements. I clamly await the cynics who will try to dismiss me as an unrepentant, boundless optimist. Optimism needs to have as much intellectual weight as witty cynicism.

"When a woman has challenges and adversities, she can rise up . . . Whoever created Gleevec, God bless them. I don't have leukemia now. My faith has the greatest emotional impact on me. The parable of the Good Samaritan was the stranger who saw the wounded man along the way, put him up on his horse, took him to the inn, and prayed for him to be cured. That is Dr. Solomon."

I think that if a thank-you gift scared him out of the room, Dr. Solomon would probably pass out if he heard this part.

Ms. Tulloch is done. She proceeds to release me.

"I know why you are writing this book," she says. "You believe that someone along the line, someone guided you on, and you were inspired by that spiritual person to write this book. There will be many more books you will be writing."

A MAN NAMED RICH has the same disease as Ms. Tulloch. He is managed in the same hospital as Ms. Tulloch. He too is taking Gleevec. Unlike Ms. Tulloch, Rich is in his early thirties and appears to be completely fit.

"I was coming in for a knee operation in 2007 for an accident," Rich says. "As a part of routine preoperative screening, they found my white cell count was very high, and they told me it looks like I might have leukemia. I had no symptoms, and that is how I found out. I would have never known."

The time between diagnosis and death in acute leukemia is from 6 to 12 weeks without treatment.

"Wow! You are so lucky!" I say.

He says nothing at first, then mumbles, "Yeah."

I ask him if he knows the name of his disease. He pauses a second, then says he doesn't know. I march cheerfully on and tell him that it's CML.

"Oh yeah, CML," he says.

"Hey," I say, "I said it first! Where you been?"

This gets a little laugh out of him.

"I figured I was going to die," he says. "They got me started on medications the same day. I started Gleevec the same day."

"So you come in, get diagnosed with leukemia, and walk out on the same day with treatment, and you have never had a symptom before or since?"

"Yup," he says. "I had a bone marrow biopsy a month ago, and they said the results are beautiful. But . . ."

Something bad is coming. There is something wrong with this man's facial expression. He looks downtrodden.

He continues, "But they want me to stay on medications anyway."

Not only is Rich's white-cell count controlled, but the very genetic derangement that caused it has been chased out of his bone marrow beyond the limits of detection. This was the last century's science fiction. Though I'm careful not to show it, his sense of entitlement and persecution makes me mad.

"Rich, you are the person this book is about," I tell him. "A few years ago, you would have either had to be transplanted or you would be dead."

It doesn't register. Instead he complains: "I have side effects."

"Like what?"

"A loss of appetite."

"Have you lost weight?"

"No, I have gained weight."

"Then I guess it is not much of a loss of appetite."

I am a persistent guy. If he's not going to levitate, quake with happiness, or express gratitude, I'd at least like to wipe the snotty persecuted look from his face. "You have been saved. But what have you been saved for?" I know I'm out of line. I just can't believe this guy dodged a bullet and never even noticed it whizzing by his ear.

"There is a purpose, but I haven't found it yet," he says.

"You have a duty to find your purpose, now that you have a life restored to you."

He mumbles a little. He tells me that he skips his medications sometimes. He has children he has not seen in two years. The only clear thing he says is: "It's an uphill battle."

I suppose that is how he sees it.

"I do feel fortunate that I have a good team of doctors that are on my side," he admits. "They made sure I got treated right away."

I try my last shot: "See, there are miracles happening around you all the time, and you don't even know it."

He shrugs his shoulders with no particular facial expression and gives a slight "Uh-huh."

I think I might have gotten through to him.

As we finish, he says, "So, when you write this book, I'm gonna get some money out of that right? Now, that might be the purpose of it all, getting some money out of this."

So much for my attempt to get him to realize the magnificence of his luck. Rich is unaware, and he likes it that way. His ignorance gives him license to be ungrateful. Contrary to what physicians who dismiss patient empowerment might believe, it is the unempowered, ignorant patient who lacks respect for his caregivers. Rich takes everything for granted and sees even a once-a-day pill as an inconvenience. His profound ingratitude and blithe blindness to the most basic facts of his own life put me into a little existential crisis. Ms. Tulloch made me feel wonderful, important, appreciated. But Rich is more useful to me. Rich compels me to have a bigger heart, to meet a higher degree of calling, to struggle to do good to people who will never thank me, never show appreciation, and never question their behavior.

I'm offended on behalf of my profession by Rich's attitude, but I also know that we must do better in communicating such blessings as his to the public.

MARTHA TUCKER IS a lovely, poised 79-year-old woman. She has a calm, measured way of speaking. Several years ago, Ms. Tucker had low back pain. Her doctor told her she had a slipped disc and sent her to physical therapy. In fact she had lymphoma—a solid collection of cancerous lymphatic cells. Improvements in the care of localized disease such as this are fantastic. Local Hodgkin's disease can be cured in 90 to 95 percent of cases usually based on radiation alone. Hodgkin's disease is cancer of the lymphatic system. The glands explode in size till they consume the entire body. In 1997, as part of the new wave of targeted therapies, researchers developed a monoclonal antibody that removes the CD20 type of lymphocytes; the specific cell that causes this cancer. If you have a drug targeted to eliminate only the cancer cell, you will leave the normal cells alone. The drug is called rituximab. There is an additional 15 percent response when it is added on top of conventional chemotherapy. That means you have to treat only seven people to get one really clear extra response.

Ms. Tucker has non-Hodgkin's lymphoma, another type of lymphatic cancer, and is treated with chemotherapy and rituximab. She has a fantastic response and has been cancer free for several years. Although misdiagnosed and clearly victimized by poor communication on the part of her doctor, she is not angry or resentful.

To be sure, I press her on the subject, but she only confirms her graciousness by saying, "Yes, I think there was some incompetence there, and this did have some effect on my trust for doctors."

I ask, "If the doctor makes a mistake like this, should the doctor apologize?"

She says, "Yes, it would be better if the doctor admitted he made a mistake. They are human, they are not perfect. But if they admit they make a mistake, it makes them more human. They can be forgiven. They can be forgiven faster if they admit they make a mistake."

Today, Ms. Tucker helps the doctor change a mistake into an opportunity for more open communication with patients.

"It doesn't help our level of trust, but it is better to confront it directly," she says. "The doctor is not God. We don't expect that."

What Ms. Tucker does expect is to be informed.

"I would just like to be talked to a little more," she says. "I did not know I was going to be half dead for a few days. I would have felt more comfortable just knowing what would happen. It was the not knowing that was difficult."

I have often wondered why people paid such high fees to the great

19th-century physician Sir William Osler, given how few tests he did and the near absence of treatments. Ms. Tucker gives the answer: accurate diagnosis and being told what to expect.

"Just give me some understanding of what will happen," she says. "Explain things to me. I had some neuropathy from the chemotherapy. I am not a child. I do not expect there to be no complications. I told them, 'I'm a big girl, just tell me what to expect. I can handle it.'"

Ms. Tucker is grateful for her cure. Although she does not understand how it works, she knows she had rituximab and that it helped control her disease. The only thing she missed was more communication.

Her daughter Bridget asks of the profession: "Just make us more of a partner in the care, for both the good and bad things that will happen. Empower us to participate with you in our care. This will make the doctor's life easier as well."

I HAD A WOMAN in the office who I have been taking care of for years. She diagnosed herself, correctly, as having irritable bowel syndrome. She had seen an advertisement for Zelnorm, a new drug at the time, known generically as tegaserod. I thought to myself, *Who are you to tell me what to prescribe? Mind your place!*

Of course, I was caught in an embarrassing mistake. In a moment of spontaneous good judgment, I had enough sense to actually say: "That is a great idea! I am so glad you brought that up. Would you like to try it and see if it works for you?"

We tried it. Her abdominal pain went away, and she sent me a valentine. Literally. I asked her why she kept coming to see me after all these years since I had so many faults: I am often late, I interrupted her, I didn't let her finish her sentences.

She said, "Because you always listen."

We are telling medical students that the profession is lesser because patients come in saying, "I read about this drug on the Internet. Can I have it?" If the medication is legitimate, patients feel great when the doctor listens to their request. They feel they have an educated, caring partner in their treatment.

Cancer patient Pauline Gordon (see chapter 21) explains it this way: "Being better educated actually helps you have a better relationship with your doctor. I am grateful for them and their help." She is clear that knowing all about her disease and treatments does not impair her sense of trust in her doctor. She sees educating herself as improving her relationship with her doctor, because it makes it easier for the doctor to educate her about side effects and treatments. "Knowing more about my disease helps my trust in my doctor because I know everything they are doing is correct. When I read about the right treatment that is supposed to be done, and then they tell me what they will do, it makes me trust them more, because I know they are right. It relaxes me."

The paradigm of the doctor-patient relationship is shifting toward partnership. The physicians among us need not only to adjust to that fact but recognize that a deep satisfaction comes with partnership. It is an enhancement, not a diminishment.

I AM AT KINGS COUNTY HOSPITAL, reviewing with a student the case of a kidney cancer patient.

The student says, "Oncology says there is no chemotherapy and to refer the patient for nephrectomy. I am discharging the patient, and she will have her kidney removed in a week or two, okay?"

"How do you know there is no chemotherapy?" I ask.

"Because oncology says so," the student responds.

I don't know if this is intellectual passivity, faith in subspecialists, or lack of time to double-check. Personally, I have a contrarian nature that says "Trust no one." I direct the student to the website ClinicalTrials. gov, a service of the U.S. National Institutes of Health.

"What's that?" she asks, like nearly every other student. Clinical-Trials.gov is a terrific tool that empowers both patients and their physicians. It makes anyone an instant cutting-edge expert. Go to www.clinicaltrials.gov and simply type in the type of cancer you're dealing with and hit Return. You get an instant list of every clinical trial in the country, if not the world, for the disease. You can search by state. You can search based on whether you have been extensively treated or not treated at all. It puts the patient in the driver's seat and allows her to have a more meaningful discussion with her doctor. Also, I am sorry to say that we caregivers cannot always be counted on to be current on every form of therapy, partly owing to the explosion of new treatments.

The student and I go on the website. There are over 1,000 trials involving kidney cancer. Over 400 of them are actively recruiting patients, and 78 of those are in New York State, where we work.

The student's eyes go wide like saucers. "Wow! I had no idea there was so much open investigation!"

I explain, "Patients are not equipped to find these studies. Patients, like you, assume that their caregiver is giving them all the options. Maybe they don't want to be in a trial, maybe they do. Your job is not to decide for them. Your job is to give them the options and let them decide. You won't diminish yourself if you think of yourself a bit like a waiter. Tell them what today's specials are, and let them decide. I am specifically not going to tell the patient the options—you are. You better be right. Her life may depend on it. "

By the next morning, the student has shown printouts of ten studies to the patient. The student is now giddy with excitement.

"She has chosen three or four she wants to look into," the student says. "I made some appointments for her and she seems much happier to have so many choices."

Just knowing there are options can suddenly make patients feel optimistic, and an active approach to their disease helps them resolve some of their anxieties. Part of the reason for the student's happiness is that medical students often feel like they're slowing down the operation. The student was excited because she brought something to the care of the patient that no one else had. She made a difference.

Clinical trials offer another amazing benefit most trainees and many doctors never think about: access to the finest care for the uninsured. Even if the therapy under study is not effective, the care in clinical trials is so excellent, so careful, so detailed, and so systematic that the patient still benefits. Evidence suggests that the survival of patients even in the placebo end of some trials is better than routine care simply because the care is so good. Don't trust me. Go to the website PubMed (www.pubmed.gov) and see for yourself. If I were one of the 47 million uninsured and suffered from a life-threatening illness, I would do my best to be on a clinical trial—any clinical trial. Not that I find it acceptable that so many people have to submit their bodies to science just to get the care they need, but until we have health coverage for all, it's an excellent option. Many of the trials have no citizenship requirement; therefore, it might be one of the only ways for a physician to get an undocumented immigrant the care he or she needs.

What if I prescribe a therapy, but my patient goes to Clinical Trials.gov and finds something else, something possibly better? If I as a caregiver feel lesser, then the flaw is in my mind, not in my relationship with my patient. ClinicalTrials.gov has 64,000 trials in 158 countries at the present time. There are 2,700 breast cancer trials alone. I daresay that even the most well-read practitioner will not be able to keep them all in mind.

PART 7

Heroic Doctors

CHAPTER 26

Managed Scare

Doctors Go Off-Label or Patients Go Blind

B OB HAD BEEN sorting letters on the job. After 30 years in the postal service, he was a few months from retirement. Bob's hobby was to paint. *Hobby* is too mild a word. Painting was Bob's meditation, his refuge, his peace. As a lifelong bachelor with no children, he has channeled all of his creative, procreative, and romantic powers through his painting. Bob's dream was to paint all day long. The problem was, Bob had been having some blurry vision. His general doctor referred him to an ophthalmologist. In short order, on a single visit, 12 minutes later, a very professional and courteous young lady informed Bob he had something called macular degeneration.

"What's that?" asked Bob, not so sure he wanted to know the answer.

No matter how slowly the doctor actually spoke, the information drenched him with the immediacy of ice water.

"Macular degeneration," the doctor said, "means the center of the back of your eye, the retina, the part that perceives light, is, well, for lack of a better word . . . dying. I am so sorry."

Macular degeneration is the most common cause of blindness in adults. It starts with central vision and proceeds inexorably to peripheral vision.

Bob asked, "When can I start treatment to reverse it?"

"That's a problem," the doctor said, then asked, "What sort of work do you do?"

"I work for the post office. I sort mail."

"Well, I am so very sorry, but at least you will have good disability coverage."

"But, doctor, I'm a painter. I've waited thirty years to do it full time. It is the thing I love most in the world. How long do I have?"

"A few months."

Bob felt like he was falling, but he knew he was still in the chair. He heard people talking to him and explaining it twice, but now he can't recall a single word of it. It wasn't just his vision becoming blurry. The whole world clouded over, and his whole life receded from view. He wondered, *What will I live for?* He didn't want to show emotion to people he'd just met in the office, but he didn't feel anything anyway.

Two days later, something happened. He got a call from the eye specialist.

"Bob, could you come in and see me tomorrow?" the specialist asked. "I have something special I want to tell you about. Something for your condition that you are going to like."

The words were like a rope coming out of the ceiling. Bob didn't have enough life left in him to say anything but that he'd be there the next day.

"We have something new," the specialist said. "It's called ranibizumab. It's a medication for your eye. Nothing like it has ever existed before. It will stop your disease."

"Stop?" Bob asked. "I thought you said there was nothing, that I would be blind for sure in a few months."

"This is new," the specialist repeated. "It might even make your vision better. But it will stop it for sure. You won't go blind."

WHEN BLOOD VESSELS grow abnormally in the retina, they block vision. Ranibizumab is a medication that stops the growth of blood vessels. It is a type of drug called a vascular endothelial growth factor (VEGF) inhibitor. (*Vascular* refers to blood vessels. *Endothelial* refers to the thin layer of cells that line some parts of the body.) In cancer, VEGF inhibitors starve the tumor. In macular degeneration, they stop the progression of disease by preventing abnormal growth of the retina. Ranibizumab stops the progression of macular degeneration in 97 percent of patients. In one-third of patients, it actually restores part of the eyesight.

The news was so unbelievable to Bob that it took a day or two to sink in.

"It was like getting a death sentence and then getting resurrected," he says.

Bob would never have described himself as a religious man. But at that moment he thought, *This is a miracle! My eyes are being restored. Sight to the blind.*

He says, "The only odd thing is, I can't recall any act of faith I ever had that would have deserved such a reward. Actually, the opposite. I thought I was doomed. I felt even too numb to think about killing myself, but I knew that would have gone through my mind."

Bob is retired now.

"Are you painting all day long like you planned?" I ask him.

"No, not as much as I thought."

Uh-oh! Trouble in paradise! I almost cannot bear to ask: "Is it your eyes?"

"No," he says. "The eyes are better than they were; not perfect, but I see all I need to. I can paint all I want, but that's not the issue."

"What happened?"

"Love."

Huh?

"I met a very nice lady in my last month on the job. She is very nice to me." Bob breaks eye contact so he can smile.

I swear I hear birds singing, but I am in an inside office with no windows. My whole day brightens up.

DR. ERIC SHRIER (see chapter 15) is a specialist in the retina. He operates through needles.

"Everything has changed to be much less invasive than it used to be since I got started in retinal surgery, and I am not that old," he says. "Everything has become minimally invasive."

Ranibizumab is injected directly into the eye, with a needle so small that you barely feel it.

Dr. Shrier says, "The coolest thing in retina medicine compared with three or four years ago is the management of macular degeneration. The VEGF inhibitors have been revolutionary. Macular degeneration was a pretty dreadful disease prior to VEGF drugs. Ninety percent of patients had at least minimal vision loss, and most had much worse vision than that. If you look at the natural history of it, macular degeneration is a blinding disease."

I tell Dr. Shrier I think it is very strange that I did not see VEGF on the six o'clock news. Fifty years ago, major medical advances were front-page news. Now we have a cure for the most common cause of blindness in the United States, and I find out about it in a one-page summary in the *Medical Letter on Drugs and Theraputics*. In the mainstream medical literature, you could easily miss the advance.

DR. RICHARD LOPEZ (see chapter 15) is an ophthalmologist who understands the immensity of what he is able to do for people, and he is able to communicate it.

"We had no answer to macular degeneration for many years," Dr. Lopez says. "People would first lose the ability to read and drive and then to negotiate around a room. I feel certain that these drugs will make it so that macular degeneration is no longer the leading cause of blindness in adults. The drug is not getting the attention it should. People are doing so well. I had a patient who lost vision in one eye from macular degeneration, then started to get it in the other eye, but now we had the VEGF drugs. She is a piano teacher. Her vision is maintained at 20/25 with monthly injections. She is still able to teach piano, to see the keys, to record and make music, which she otherwise before would not have been able to do. People who would have inevitably gone blind are now maintained. I injected ten people just today. I graduated from my residency in 1983, but this is the best thing since the invention of the laser in the 1970s. I can't tell you how exciting it is."

VEGF inhibitors were not created for eye diseases. They were first developed to fight cancer. Bevacizumab (manufactured under the brand name Avastin), the first major drug in the class, was developed for metastatic colon cancer, which it fights very well. It is only since 2004 that VEGF inhibitors have been used for macular degeneration. Ranibizumab was approved in 2006.

DR. SHRIER IS QUICK to point out that he has been using Avastin for a number of diseases besides macular degeneration, including neovascular glaucoma. Glaucoma is a disease of the hypertension of the eyeball. In a healthy eye, the fluid inside, or aqueous humor, drains out of a passage called the canal of Schlemm. If the canal is blocked, the accumulation of fluid starts to put pressure on the optic nerve. Over time, the pressure destroys the optic nerve and the patient goes blind. In neovascular glaucoma, abnormal new blood vessels form that clog the canal of Schlemm. Avastin stops the growth of the blood vessels, opens the canal, and reverses the disease.

Dr. Shrier has also used VEGF inhibitors for retinal vein occlusion, a painless, sudden blockage of the flow of blood out of the eye, which prior to VEGF drugs meant the patient just went blind. He has also used them to treat the overgrowth of blood vessels in the eye called diabetic retinopathy. The standard therapy is to control blood sugar levels and to apply a laser to the back of the eye. Sometimes the laser treatment fails. Now there is at least an alternative treatment.

Dr. Lopez adds, "One of the biggest reasons VEGF drugs are so important is in the treatment of people in underserved areas. I have worked in the middle of reservations when there was no electricity and no laser. People have been maintained by my going out there every few weeks or months and just injecting them. The drug does not get the attention it deserves."

Dr. Shrier is quick to point out that these are off-label uses of the drugs. *Off-label* means that, according to the package insert—the sheet of paper enclosed with a medication that is the official description of what the drug is, how it works, and what it is good for—the drug is not approved for a particular use. It is essentially a legal document that includes precise indications for which the drug is specifically approved.

Whenever a physician uses a drug without a specific FDA-approved indication, he puts himself a risk. If the procedure does not go well, the patient can turn around and crucify him for doing something not specifically approved in the package insert. The physician may be able to point to evidence in a journal to justify his work, but that won't stand up to the clearly justifiable uses included by the FDA. Another risk is that insurance companies do not like physicians to do treatments without proven evidence. That is good. Protect the patient from quacks, incompetents, and weirdos who want to do a treatment that is not part of the FDA-approved list. The insurance company wants to keep us mad scientists from doing bad things to patients with crazy, unapproved therapies, so, if it is not an approved indication, they do not pay.

Sure, sure. I can see the good in that. Insurers should refuse to reimburse people who are going blind to protect them from last-ditch efforts. Good thing insurance companies are fighting to protect us from our doctors' treatment plans. After all, doctors turn to off-label uses only for a self-serving interest in, uh . . . Hmm. I guess this argument does not figure. Doctors do not work on commission for medications used. Off-label use accrues liability risk. A doctor using a medication off-label is putting his license on the line to provide the patient with a chance at not going blind.

We physicians in general are not a risk-taking group. In fact, quite the opposite. We look at evidence and weigh options. Most of the time, our choices stem from the right reason: how can I help? Sometimes we have more cautious reasons: first do no harm. Sometimes we act from cowardice: I don't want to get sued. But, whichever way you slice it, we are in general a risk-averse group. That is good; no one wants to get hurt. On the other hand, maybe a patient has a rare disease, such as retinal vein occlusion or neovascular glaucoma, that has not accumulated a billion-dollar level of interest from a pharmaceutical company. If you are someday given a diagnosis of a disease with few treatment options, you may want to ask your doctor—after he tells you there is little he can do—whether there any unapproved therapies without clear evidence that he can at least try. Let him off the hook. Tell him, "I will not hold you responsible if I have a side effect; I just want to try something." Maybe you will find he has heard of some long-shot therapy.

I only recommend this course of action until we have a better system in place, one in which doctors are free to act according to their best judgment. Some people actually advocate making the patient the decider as a matter of policy. Explain that the drug is too new to be proven and ask patients to consent to therapy knowing it is risky. But how is a patient equipped to make a truly informed consent? Despite my own hypertrophied knowledge base, even I did not know of many of the treatments I have described in this book. I could no more make an informed decision about them than I would be able to make an informed decision about repairing a car. The mechanic is the one who understands the problem. I can get a second opinion, but at the end of the day I am dependent on someone with an area of specialized knowledge to tell me the best thing to do.

Imagine a doctor making the following statements: "Hi, Bob, how's it going at the post office? I want to use a recombinantly produced humanized monoclonal antibody fragment. It is a vascular endothelial growth factor inhibitor to retard new blood vessel growth in neovascular glaucoma. What do you think?"

Maybe Bob, in the seven minutes or so provided for physician contact in a reimbursed office visit, can learn what Dr. Shrier learned in four years of medical school, four years of residency, and two years of fellowship.

Where do physicians hold their largest meetings? There are not a lot of cities that can accommodate such a vast horde descending on them. Las Vegas is a city that can. But most physicians' meetings are not held there. It has to do with the fundamental nature of physicians: we don't gamble. We look at the gaming tables and know we will have to lose eventually. That's the odds. The P value of statistical probability is set against us. We know the casino is raking in dough. We know that the games favor the house. The core of our scientific reasoning is this: do not believe your senses; look at the evidence. No amount of flashing lights and spilling of slot machine money in a bin is going to make us participate in gambling. The belief that luck will beat the odds is simply not in our worldview.

If you want your hyperrational, nongambling doctor to try an off-label use of a drug, you'd better be sure to ask him for it specifically. And be sure you make him understand that you know it is a gamble.

DR. SHRIER IS THE Clark Kent of our story—a mild-mannered retina surgeon at the top of his game who at a moment's notice does something heroic. Every time he makes an off-label prescription, in a thoughtful, well-considered effort to help when there is no other help, he places himself at risk of criticism and legal repercussions. On the other hand, insurance companies are most often for-profit businesses, with stockholders and high CEO compensation. The more money they save on treatments, the more money they have to distribute to the owners and operators of the company. Consequently, they often refuse to pay for treatment not considered to be the standard of care. Here is the statement: "Doctor, we don't tell you how to practice medicine; we just tell you what we will pay for."

The wholesale cost of a 4-milliliter vial of Avastin is $687. This makes it considerably more expensive than gold. An ounce is 28 grams. 28 grams of Avastin costs $252,000. That would be wholesale, of course, not counting a 20 percent markup for the retailer.

Across the board, doctors and students identify dealing with health insurance companies as problematic. The number one, least satisfying, most painful experience for physicians is dealing with health insurance companies. Ninety-two percent of physicians and students agreed or strongly agreed that dealing with insurance companies made medicine less satisfying and less attractive to practice. Seven percent were "neutral." Put another way, only 1 percent of physicians did *not* feel that the single greatest source of dissatisfaction in medicine was the health insurance industry and the complexity and pain of the system of working with them.

We *must* make medicine more satisfying and attractive for those people.

When asked, If you did *not* have to work for a living, would you still practice medicine, 80 percent of respondents said they would still practice medicine.

Health insurers have a vested interest in keeping the system of reimbursement the same. Their profits are based on health care rationing and denial of payments.

You wait and see the next time a push is made for universal coverage. The health insurance industry will pour unlimited amounts of money into advertising to scare you. The socialized medicine monster will come out of the closet. Part of its propaganda is that universal coverage will eliminate "choice." Right now, your physician does not have the choice to use treatments for you if your insurance company claims they are experimental. Where is the choice in that? If your physician wants to hospitalize you for better care, the insurer can deny payment because it did not agree with your physician's judgment that this was best for you. Where is the choice in that? If your physician wants to keep you in the hospital for an extra day's observation, the insurer will have its reviewer send the doctor a notice saying "Coverage denied." Then you, the patient, will have to pay. Where is the choice in that?

The health insurance industry will do everything it can to keep the system the way it is now. Unlimited CEO compensation, denial of coverage for medications, denial of coverage for hospitalization, an excruciating preapproval process for medications and procedures. The single greatest obstacle to freedom of action is the insurance industry.

Many successful treatments get their start as off-label drugs. This is partly because it is hard to accumulate sufficient data on rare diseases, such as retinal vein occlusion. A new indication (a new use for which the drug may be indicated) can cost upward of $100 million to obtain, even for a drug already approved. This is the amount of money it takes to design, review, and implement the studies necessary to obtain FDA approval of the new indication. A drug company is not likely to start the process without evidence that it will at least make its money back, if not a profit.

Without an FDA-approved indication, there is another way to get insurers to pay for the drugs, but it is long and slow. Once enough doctors use a drug for a particular disease, FDA-approved or not, it becomes part of the standard of care. This is common. It is scary for any physician to go first, but in retinal vein occlusion the doctor has to act immediately to prevent blindness. In severe proliferative diabetic retinopathy unresponsive to laser photocoagulation, the patient will go blind before the data can accumulate. Under managed care, there are these two choices: the uncertainty of going off-label or the certainty of going blind.

I would give to each of you, my brothers—you who hear me now, and to you whom may elsewhere read my words—to you who do our greatest work laboring incessantly for small rewards in towns and country places—to you the more favored ones who have special fields of work—to you teachers and professors and scientific workers—to one and all, through the length and breadth of the land—I give a single word as my parting commandment . . . CHARITY.
—Sir William Osler, "Aequanimitas," 1889

CHAPTER 27

A Battle Axe Hits a Disease

One Doctor's Fight to Change Rheumatology

To GO INTO rheumatology—the study of diseases of joints such as osteoarthritis, rheumatoid arthritis, and gout, as well as all the auto-immune diseases such lupus—either you have to be completely insensitive or you have to have a level of compassion and empathy that must be nearly excruciating. Cures are virtually nonexistent. The diseases are progressive, and almost none has fully effective therapy. Compared to oncology, rheumatology is both easy and hard. The easy part is that patients don't die. The hard part is that they slowly get worse and worse.

Most autoimmune diseases affect four to five times more women than men. The same hypervigilant immune system that guards women against heart attacks can also turn against their bodies. It is like a too-sensitive car alarm. When a truck goes by, the vibration sets off the alarm, even though the car has not been touched. This is an autoimmune disease.

I go to the rheumatology clinic for a few weeks in search of a miracle and always leave disappointed. The fellows and faculty in the division all have the blasé faces of people doing the usual. When I describe the miracles I am looking for, I get incredulous looks that say, "Have you considered psychotherapy, Conrad?"

My boss says: "Just skip them, Conrad, and concentrate on the other areas."

He is insightful about most everything, so I am about to give up the search.

As a last-ditch effort, I go to see the rheumatology division chief, Dr. Ellen Ginzler, a full professor of medicine at SUNY Downstate who has changed the standard of care in the world for lupus nephritis (kidney disease in lupus). Dr. Ginzler has a reputation for being demanding and angry—but no wonder: her job could be a case study in frustration. I ask her about the biggest breakthroughs in rheumatology. What I hear is not poetic.

She points out, "Almost all the drugs used in lupus have been borrowed from other areas in medicine like oncology or drugs to prevent transplant rejection. It has been forty years since the approval of the last new drug specifically for lupus."

Dr. Ginzler figured out how to more effectively control the T cells at the root of the problem with a treatment that causes fewer side effects than previous treatments. Physicians used to rely on steroids and an immunosuppressive drug called cyclophosphamide; because of Dr. Ginzler's efforts, we now use steroids and a medication called mycophenolate mofetil. Mycophenolate is an immunosuppressive drug that stops the proliferation of the T cell.

With justified frustration, Dr. Ginzler says, "I could not get the manufacturer interested in studying this drug. I could not get anyone in a meaningful position of authority there to pick it up."

Dr. Ginzler is a well-published clinician-scientist who is smart, stalwart, and aggressive.

She continues: "Mycophenolate was approved in 1995 for organ transplant rejection. We thought it was reasonable to study it for lupus nephritis, but all that was being presented were small case series and individual reports. It wasn't good enough to convince the FDA or the manufacturer to fund a study. I had been trying desperately to get the manufacturer to fund the study. All it was was $200,000 a year for three years. That is not a lot of money to run a multicenter study. I couldn't even find anyone who would even talk to me. I found out later the reason for this was that they were studying mycophenolate for rheumatoid arthritis and it was going very badly. They chose very sick rheumatoid arthritis patients, and it wasn't working. I went back again, and again. I rewrote the grant. At the last minute, they decided to give me the drug, and I got funded. The entire funding for the project was $600,000 from the FDA and $250,000 from the drug company. This is a very small amount of money for a large drug company."

In other words, through her perseverance, Dr. Ginzler managed to ram through the study.

The drug industry often fails creative clinician-scientists. It is an institution devoted to profits, not cures. That is why there are multiple new drugs for erectile dysfunction but barely anything new for malaria. There are millions of Americans with cash looking for a better erection. The people dying of malaria live in places without this kind of money. Physicians must do double time in having to work the system; many of them are going to heroic lengths to get their patients the care they need. I have spoken with many strong doctors who aren't waiting for the insurance and drug industries to do the right thing but are instead taking matters into their own hands. I hope the day will come soon that physicians don't have to be superheroes just to get their patients the medications and procedures they need, because the fight is wearing down the spirits of physicians across the profession. But until that day, physicians and patients alike can be grateful and hopeful that there are Ellen Ginzlers in the world.

Dr. Ginzler comes across as an M1 tank to many of her colleagues. I have many times sat in a faculty meeting or watched her bark at the chairperson in a division chiefs meeting. Her tone is the harshest I know in the medical school. Sometimes she is angry on behalf of her patients, for whom she shows tremendous compassion. Her success in changing the standard of care in lupus nephritis means that fewer patients are in need of kidney transplants—which is especially significant, since there are not nearly enough kidneys available for all the people who need transplants. The prevention or delay of kidney disease in lupus patients also mercifully keeps them off dialysis. Preventing death on a transplant list is a miracle. Dr. Ginzler has made it routine. She is a hero to thousands of men and women who suffer from lupus nephritis and their loved ones.

DR. GINZLER INVITES me to the clinic where she sees patients and supervises the care. A patient comes by. Ellen enfolds the young woman in her left arm and starts to talk with me about the drugs that have kept her lupus stable. She brings me into the room of a man with an auto-immune disease. She is transformed. I am bowled over by her warmth, kindness, and compassion. Another patient comes in.

Dr. Ginzler says, "Oh, come and talk to her! Isn't she adorable? Isn't she beautiful? Let me tell you about what we have done for her."

Suddenly I see how deeply this doctor cares about the people she is responsible for. In the face of incurable diseases that are among the most frustrating in all of medicine, I see patients coming for relief to this oasis of warmth and goodwill. Dr. Ginzler inhales fear and anxiety, and exhales concern and consideration.

She is now a bundle of energy. She whisks me into a room to meet Ms. Doris Frost, who suffers from rheumatoid arthritis.

"Here is the type of patient you have been wanting to see," Dr. Ginzler says. "Talk to her for a while."

Ms. Frost is 65 years old and is best described as a nice church lady.

"When I first came here to the rheumatology clinic in 1993," she says, "my son had to carry me in here. I could barely walk."

In the medical community, rheumatoid arthritis is a so-called bad disease, meaning a progressive disease of unknown cause. For bad diseases, treatments are not fully effective and often painful; moreover, the treatments may have dangerous side effects.

Ms. Frost is friendly, small, kindhearted, and long-suffering.

"I am a very spiritual person," she says. "My faith is the strongest thing in my life. I love God. I love my church. I was just praying to feel better. I prayed to God, but I couldn't get into it like I wanted to. I was a waitress when I was still working. First I would drop the heavy things. Then I couldn't even hold on to a plate. I would drop it because I couldn't close my hand. I got depressed, and I started to use antidepressants like Prozac and Zoloft. If you don't feel good, you can't concentrate."

Ms. Frost suffered the kind of soul-withering debility that melts away hope. Rheumatoid arthritis has no cure. And it is not rare. Nearly 1 percent of the U.S. population has rheumatoid arthritis. One percent means nearly 2.1 million people. Many people do not know anyone who has rheumatoid arthritis; that is possibly because people with rheumatoid arthritis become invisible as the disease progresses. They withdraw from life; their world becomes narrow. They are tired, so they stay home. They are anemic, so they don't go out and participate as much. Maybe someone at your workplace has rheumatoid arthritis, but you may not realize it until she disappears from work one day to go out on disability. Rheumatoid arthritis saps life from the patient over time and doesn't arouse the immediate emotional response people give to cancer or a heart attack. Rheumatoid arthritis is not a fatal disease, so to speak. It doesn't have angry young political activists as AIDS does. There are no pink ribbons as in breast cancer. Our reminders of people suffering from rheumatoid arthritis are only as obvious as a plate dropping in a restaurant. It might be the next Doris Frost whose joints are so deformed that she cannot close her hand.

Thanks to the translation of rheumatologists' anger into action, Ms. Frost has gotten adalimumab (manufactured under the brand name Humira) for the last few years. Adalimubab, approved for use in 2003, is a laboratory-generated biological agent (see chapter 23). It is a mediator of immunity and activator of an entire cascade of white blood cells that attack normal joint tissue.

"I have been on Humira for three years," Ms. Frost says. "Nothing before worked. I couldn't walk. Methotrexate did not do that much for me."

I ask her what it's like now.

"I can do everything," she replies. "All my stiffness and inflammation got so much better. Now I can move. My hands use to swell up; now they don't. I don't have as much pain. I feel better. I am more cheerful. I am less angry. My faith is the strongest thing in my life. I prayed to feel better. Now I can pray for other things because I feel better. I used to feel crippled. Now I can worship."

I am still skeptical and ask her what she can do now that she couldn't do before the Humira.

"I can go to the gym," she says.

My eyes bulge out of my head. "Are you serious?"

A woman who had to be carried into the doctor's office and couldn't carry something as light as a plate for 10 years is now going to the gym! A person with rheumatoid arthritis for 15 years is now on the treadmill lifting weights.

"I feel like God sent Humira to me," Ms. Frost continues. "You pray for help. You pray to feel better. To bring me something to make me feel better." Her tone is plaintive and strained. Her voice is trying like a weight lifter to push an immovable weight. "I was very depressed, let me put it that way. When I was on the other medicine, it didn't do much for me. Humira was the only thing that really helped me. Now I don't take Zoloft or Prozac anymore. I don't take any of that anymore. I don't know if you can understand. I threw away my antidepressant medications."

"What effect did your disease have on your relationships?" I ask.

"Well, my children are all grown, so that wasn't the problem. They had their own life, so it didn't affect them that much."

"Did you have a man in your life?"

"Oh no! I couldn't!" she answers emphatically, with a grimace and a sudden, firm shake of her head.

"Did you get one since you went on the Humira?"

"Oh yes, I have a friend," she answers very quickly with a giggle like a teenager's. "I met him in my building. He goes to church with me. He prays with me. And do you know how hard it is to find someone like that?"

I ask, "So the Humira allowed you to throw away your antidepressants, go to the gym, and get a man?"

Ms. Frost is excited now. "You know what I am so happy for? He likes me because I can move! I am not like the other sixty-five-year-old women. He likes me because I am so active. He is my age. He likes me because I can *move*. You know I am not rich, but now I am rich in other things."

Ms. Frost acknowledges that she was doubtful at first.

"I wasn't getting much help from the other medications," she says. "I didn't want to try Humira at first. But look at my fingers now. See how they are straight? . . . My fingers straightened. I couldn't move them before . . . My doctor said, 'Try it,' and I tried it. If you don't feel good, you can't concentrate. You got to try things. Now I can do what I want to do."

Ms. Frost's doctor was able to open her mind and offer hope with two simple words: "try it." However, what can that doctor say to a patient with lupus, for whom there has been no major new drug approved in the last 40 years? If you were a patient facing a debilitating, painful disease. would you like your doctor to say, "Sorry, ma'am, we don't have anything much to offer you. When you have a flare we will give you steroids that, if used for more than two weeks, are associated with all sorts of nasty side effects." Or would you rather hear, "The last few years have seen amazing improvement in our treatment of rheumatoid arthritis and other diseases. There are advances in our understanding of the immune system, and new drugs are in the pipeline of development. Do not despair—hold on! Help is on the way."

Would such words have only a placebo effect? I don't think so. I think providing hope to these patients is just as critical as providing whatever relief from physical symptoms we can. People can bear almost any form of suffering as long as they know it is temporary, that someone cares, and that someone is working for a cure. There is enormous benefit for a patient with an excruciating rheumatologic disease to know that someone is working to break them out of their prison.

I once asked a field operative for Human Rights Watch what was the most dramatic things he had personally done to help someone. I was surprised to hear that it was not facilitating the release of someone unjustly imprisoned. The greatest emotional impact for her was making a first visit to someone who had been unjustly imprisoned for well over a year. The detainee began to cry upon learning that someone was out there working for his release. He was not alone, and many people were working for his freedom.

In the case of rheumatoid arthritis, which is also like being imprisoned, in that the body becomes a cage, clinician-scientists are bringing hope at a terrific rate. Consider the following list of treatments:

1950	Azulfidine	1991–1997	Nothing
1955	Plaquenil	1998	Etanercept, infliximab, leflunomide
1959	Methotrexate		
1960	Gold	2001	Anakinra
1961–1970	Nothing	2003	Adalimumab (Humira)
1971–1980	Nothing	2005	Abatacept
1981–1990	Nothing	2006	Rituximab

In the last 10 years, more drugs have been approved for use than in the last 60 years. These drugs also have fewer side effects. Telling patients that they do not have to despair is not offering false hope. It is a fact.

Most people will respond to a person with a severely deformed hand with compassion for the pain and depression wrought by the tortured joints. Most people would love to offer help and hope. Feeling compassion to the point of trying to do something about the pain is a sign of a hero. The hero asks, "What can I do to make Ms. Frost feel better?" The hero guards her compassion, is willing to bear pain for the sake of another, and does something to make it better. But the hero is not invulnerable. The hero needs help. She needs to know where we are winning. Knowing that there are routine miracles fills her tank, charges her batteries, heals her own wounds.

I want to encourage contemplation of what physicians are doing well in medicine so they will have more energy to be present to helping others more. I want us all to be angry that there are not enough cures and not enough access to care because not everyone has health insurance. I want us to be as furious as Dr. Ellen Ginzler that people have to choose between paying for their medications and paying for clothing, or a tank of gas, or sometimes even food. I want us to be furious that pain occurs that can be relieved but is not. I want us to be angry because anger creates action.

CHAPTER 28

"Medicine Is an Art"

The Legacy of Sir William Osler

WILLIAM OSLER WAS born in Canada in 1849. As the son of a minister, he too embarked on a path toward the ministry. The title *sir* would come later in life, after he had revolutionized the practice of medicine and medical education. In 1889, Osler became physician-in-chief at Johns Hopkins School of Medicine. With this move, he started the first university hospital in the United States.

"Medicine is an art, not a trade, a calling, not a business, a calling in which your heart will be exercised equally with your head," Osler wrote in his 1889 book, *Aequanimitas*. This sentence was Osler's theme. It is why he is a giant in medicine. The radiant grandeur of Osler's optimism and his reverence for students make him as relevant today as he was a century ago. By being open minded, creative, and scientific artists rather than tradesmen, doctors can find satisfaction in their work and help patients to find cures or at least a better quality of life.

Besides celebrating the sacred calling of the physician in his numerous books, papers, and addresses, Osler created the basis for training that every school and residency in the country follows today. Prior to Osler, the standard medical school curriculum took two years. Students paid faculty directly, then went straight into practice. Osler raised the standard of training by expanding the duration of medical school from two to four years. He also invented the internship and residency. Like young seminarians, doctors in training lived where they learned and worked, hence the name *residents*. The earliest residents could not be accepted if they were married. They were to have no distractions, no interests other than their work. They were to totally immerse themselves in training and to make medicine a way of life.

Prior to Osler, clinical education was haphazard. He regimented a pattern that is now considered indispensable to training. He created the clinical clerkship, a system of block rotations in the third and fourth year of medical school where students spend several months at a time in each clinical specialty: two or three months on surgery, two months on obstetrics, and two or three or four months on internal medicine. Bedside teaching was at the center of his method. Osler created the standard for training by examining the patient and discussing the case at the patient's bedside. After hearing the history, Osler made standard the now universally accepted pattern of examination of the patient: inspection, palpation, auscultation, and contemplation.

"Medicine is learned by the bedside and not in the classroom. Let not your conceptions of disease come from words heard in the lecture room or read from the book. See, and then reason and compare and control, but see first," he taught. Osler changed clinical education from a classroom to a hands-on experience. In doing so, he centered the meaning of medicine as a service and investigation of disease as it pertained to an individual suffering in the moment. He brought humanism to the science.

Osler's humanism begat the end of suffering for untold numbers of patients, not directly but by the influence it had on the scientific community and the world at large. One of Osler's first residents at Johns Hopkins was Harvey Cushing, who went on to write a Pulitzer Prize–winning biography of Osler. Less known to the general public than Osler, Cushing basically invented the field of neurosurgery. He is a towering figure in that field: nearly a dozen diseases, physical findings, and conditions are named after him. Physicians and patients alike must have difficulty imagining the strength of character it would take to be a neurosurgeon operating before the invention of the CT scan, magnetic resonance imaging, and antibiotics. His formidable innate gifts aside, Cushing was precisely the kind of student that results from teachers who encourage possibility and have faith that their charges will not only meet but exceed their greatest hopes. I shudder to think how many modern-day Harvey Cushings are dissuaded by their mentors' negative attitudes and by the insurance and drug industries' treatment of their work as a trade.

Osler achieved his widest acclaim with the publication in 1892 of *The Principles and Practice of Medicine.* The first modern textbook of medicine, it was required reading not only for physicians and medical students but for anyone who claimed to be literate in matters of the day. For more than 20 years, it was the best-selling textbook of medicine in the world. Never before had a comprehensive textbook of medicine been written covering every field of endeavor. Its main theme was Osler's belief that the primary purpose of medicine was to make diagnoses, give prognoses, and protect patients from ineffective therapy. Barely a third of the diseases he included had any form of treatment listed. Osler charged that any physician claiming to successfully treat either pneumonia or cancer must be a charlatan. In an article in *Science* magazine in 1891 he wrote, "One of the first duties of the physician is to educate the masses not to take medicine."

In an age with no "great physicians," it is difficult to imagine the esteem and regard with which Osler was held in his own day. Osler, although disparaging of politicians, was routinely physician to members of Congress and the president's cabinet. He was physician to the Astor family. His income from fees would approach a million dollars a year in today's currency. The literary luminary of Baltimore journalism of the time, H. L. Mencken, who had few kind things to say about anyone, wrote of "the curious enchantment that he [Osler] worked upon all who had any sort of contact with him." Osler had contact with many celebrities and powerful figures of his time, including Winston Churchill, Herbert Hoover, Rudyard Kipling, and Walt Whitman. At the request of King Edward, he became physician to Edward, Prince of Wales, who would later abdicate the throne to become the Duke of Windsor. Later in life, Osler turned down the opportunity to be a physician to the court of the king of England.

In the summer of 1897, a Baptist minister by the name of Frederick Gates took *The Principles and Practice of Medicine* on his summer holiday. Gates happened also to be philanthropic adviser to one John D. Rockefeller. Gates read the book cover to cover. He was impressed by two things: the quality of the book, and the fact that the majority of diseases mentioned in it had no treatment. Gates determined in a 1904 letter to Osler that America's rich must alter the course of their philanthropic gifts from religious institutions and dedicate some of their wealth to "practical applications of physical and chemical sciences."

Gates had previously advised that large-scale philanthropy be directed to the Baptist Church. He now told Rockefeller of the work of Louis Pasteur in France and advised Rockefeller to start a large-scale medical research institute in the United States. Overnight was born the first medical research institute in the country, the Rockefeller Institute for Medical Research, now known as the Rockefeller University in New York City. Osler himself had no idea of Gates's plans and had nothing to do with setting up the institute. Since 1901, scientists at the Rockefeller University have garnered 23 Nobel Prizes. Full of hope and faith in the power of science to end human suffering, Osler wrote a book, and those who had ears to hear set up the greatest private research powerhouse in the country.

I am certain that if Osler were alive today, he would be enraptured by all we have to offer patients. Yes, it is true that there are 47 million uninsured people in the United States, but Osler would look at it from the point of view that 85 percent of the population does have insurance, whereas in his time there was none. Osler would think it a magnificent thing that there is a statutory mandate to provide emergency care to everyone, regardless of ability to pay. Osler would be grateful for a universally safe water supply, never mind the explosion of mortality-lowering therapeutics. He would be astounded to learn of a catheter shaped like a corkscrew that can snatch a clot from the human brain in order to restore blood flow and reverse a stroke; a probe that can be inserted into a huge cancer in the liver and essentially melt the tumor; a scope that uses the body's natural orifices to give physicians access to points inside the human body with no incision. He would be pleased to see his textbook replaced by a system of medical subspecialization so vast that physicians in one area can hardly keep up with advances in another.

Osler is without peer in combining poetry and practicality to describe the lifelong learner. He will never be forgotten as long as humanity seeks light, hope, and the power of optimism. It is the radiant power of optimism to dissolve all obstacles, to right all wrongs, to transform suffering into comfort despite any difficulty that this book is about. There is enormous goodness, triumph, and success pouring out of medicine at the present moment, but we are not capturing the emotional power of our own success to conquer the next disease, the next obstacle. Medical students have never been better trained than now. The size of the faculty at medical schools has never been larger. The ability to heal, cure, and relieve suffering has never been better than now. If a century ago Osler could write in "Aequanimitas," "The average sum of human suffering has been reduced in a way to make the angels rejoice," one can only imagine what he would say today.

WHEN I WAS at the end of my internship, I experienced, as interns often do, a period of despondency about my purpose as a physician. I was far enough along to have a basic competence, but my work was deficient in meaning. Patients were problems to be handled. Lab tests were data points, and treatments were managed with less depth than orders in a fast-food joint. I was not held to be less sensitive than the other residents. In fact, it was expected and even routine for physicians in training to have a kind of burnt-out cynicism and emotional opacity. When I broached the subject, even kindly older physicians would shrug. They seemed sympathetic toward my suffering, but they were not concerned about my crisis of faith. Internship was expected to be difficult and routine to the point of being desensitizing.

One faculty member who was more kindly than the rest said, "Don't worry, you will get your sensitivity back; it comes back when you are done with residency." But even this statement implied that I was not expected to be too caring. Still, my conscience called to me in quiet moments just loudly enough to make me know that I was missing something.

I set myself a task to talk to ten physicians I respected to find out what they loved most about medicine. For some, it was the long-term relationship with people who were depending on them. For some, it was the opportunity to open a clogged artery and to know that heart was fed by blood better than before. Others, unfortunately, seemed to be just as clueless as I was, but they were able to perform well through practice and because they were fundamentally honorable people. My last stop was my favorite teacher, Greg Steinberg, a master in bedside teaching and a jovial, warm man whose jet-black hair made him look ten years younger than he was. When I told him that I felt insufficient meaning in my daily work, he was quick to respond.

"Osler!" he said. "Go find Sir William, and he will have what you need."

I set out that very evening to the medical library at Columbia University. I easily found many works by Sir William Osler in the catalog, but when I went to look in the stacks, they were in the farthest reaches of the bottom floor of a library five stories underground. I was on an archeological dig! On the last day of my quest, with the last of my ten chosen doctors, I felt something meaningful was finally coming my way. I opened a book not taken out for over 50 years. Perhaps I am given to magical thinking, but I felt that these books were waiting for me to rescue them from the oblivion of obscurity. I opened the first one to drop into my hand, *Counsels and Ideals*. My eyes fell upon the line "Happiness lies in the absorption in some vocation which satisfies the soul." My life changed on the spot. A feeling of purpose flooded into me. My internship was no longer some mechanical, backbreaking indoctrination into medicine. The man who designed the form of training that I was in every day had never intended it that way.

I AM REMINDED of my own pre-Oslerian despair by what seems at times to be an army of negative physicians, faculty members, and, I am sorry to say, role models for students.

A 2008 Gallup survey shows public trust of physicians at an all-time high, but 80 percent of students and doctors can't believe it. I ask medical students who were toddlers 25 years ago whether it was better to practice then, and nearly everyone insists that it was. With small exception, the advances in this book are treatments available only within the last 25 years, yet medical professionals sweep that away as somehow beside the point. In 1905, Osler warned students, "Some will tell you that the profession is under-rated, unhonored, underpaid, its members social drudges—the very last profession they would recommend a young person to take up. Listen not to these croakers. The evils they deprecate lie in themselves."

The profession has adopted evidence-based medicine as the cornerstone of its educational system for practice and care, yet the most critical feature of evidence-based medicine must include physicians' examination of their own minds. How, based on the evidence that we can do more now than ever for a suffering humanity, can anyone claim that this is not the best time in history to be in medicine?

It is time for a renaissance of the physician's spirit. From within the profession, faculty can enlighten and encourage students and themselves by concentrating on all the good they are able to do. Faculty can cease bemoaning the "weakness" or the perceived lack of commitment of students and residents and fully project positivity, encouragement, and breathless excitement that *this* is the best time ever to be in medicine and that *now* we are a hair's breadth from the breakthroughs and cures that healers have sought for millennia. Now is the time, and these students are the ones that can do it. Faculty members can do their part by insisting that students pass them and do better than they did. From outside the profession, government and society can do their part by removing the oppressive system of managed care, granting universal health coverage, and seeing that potential new treatments get the funding they need.

In 1902, before the invention of almost all forms of treatment we now use, Osler wrote: "Never has the outlook for the profession been brighter. Everywhere the physician is better trained and better equipped than he was twenty-five years ago. Disease is understood more thoroughly, studied more carefully, and treated more skillfully." More than a century later, medicine requires not so much a healer for the art of medicine itself but a fighter. This age needs steel-spined, courageous, and optimistic warriors in medicine. The fight is to achieve universal health care despite an army of third-party insurers entrenched behind battlements of fixed ideas, self-interest, greed, and lack of political will. The fight is against, I regret, senior physicians and thought leaders who corrupt the minds of the next generation of physicians with nostalgia for an outmoded past. The fight is to never accept anyone in medicine who—by word, facial expression, or stifled groan—leads our students to believe anything except that they are the most knowledgeable, best trained, most capable generation ever to exit a medical school. The fight is to never accept anyone in medicine who offers a patient false despair.

The fight is to look up, like Osler, Cushing, Gates, and Rockefeller, toward what we can do, not down at what we haven't done. Perhaps part of physician dissatisfaction in medicine is from a lack of goals, now that so many have been met. I believe that a key to rekindling our passion is to raise our expectations. I believe we can capture both the public's and the profession's imagination by raising expectations to measurable lofty goals, such as the cure of diabetes. Osler's ideas can bring energy that is not only inexhaustible but also self-renewing to the medical profession. As a long as there is one person striving to serve a suffering humanity, there will be a chain reaction of hope on contact with his or her ideas.

Osler's biography is not as important as the immortality of his ideas on work and study. He championed lifelong learning, charity, and devotion to medicine as a way of life. It is not the amount of work physicians do that creates happiness; it is the amount of meaning derived from the work. What Osler teaches is that the relief of pain and the discovery of new treatments that provide hope for patients can bring fulfillment to the lives of practitioners.

We are . . . doing amazing things with scoliosis surgery. We replace discs.
That did not exist before. I was thinking about how the only job these kids
would be qualified for in the Middle Ages would be a court jester. All they
would have been ready for was to swing on a rope around Notre Dame.
You take a deformed twisted kid with scoliosis and untwist them. They get
stretched out. You can't imagine how deformed these kids were. These kids
[were] twisted before surgery, and they are straight afterward.
  —Dr. Bill Urban, chair of orthopedics, SUNY Downstate

EPILOGUE

IT'S A LUCKY DAY for me. I have an urgent spine case to discuss, and I find two experts in the same room at the same time. Dr. Michael Gerling, the director of spine surgery at the State University Health Sciences Center at Brooklyn, happens to be in the office of Dr. Steve Onesti, the chair of neurosurgery. Spine surgery is somewhere in between neurosurgery and orthopedics, depending on the case. The orthopedist handles the bone around the spine, and the neurosurgeon handles the meat in between.

"Hold on a second," I say. "I'll run and get the films."

I grab both the X-rays and spinal CT scan and run back to show them. The room is heady with expertise. I inhale all the powerful IQ. When I am with Steve Onesti, I joke about every little problem with "Hey, it's not brain surgery! Oh. Actually, in your case, it *is* brain surgery!" He doesn't find it funny, at least not after the fifth time.

"Give me a sentence on the case," Dr. Gerling says. He has the chiseled good looks of a soap opera star playing a doctor or a movie star who always plays the hero, only he is the real deal. I believe heroes are essential to a properly functioning society. We need to have people to look up to and admire. Not in the sense of "They are better than I am," but rather in the spirit of "I want to grow, I want to be a hero, I want to conquer evil and make the world a better place, so I want to be near people who inspire me."

The goal of medicine is the relief of suffering and the elimination of disease. Seek an environment where you are inspired by the local heroes, and simultaneously struggle to be good enough to be a hero for others. Everyone simultaneously being inspired and inspiring others. Everyone moves up, everyone grows. Our growth conquers ignorance and creates new methods and treatments. This results in the healing of an individual as well as improving the art of healing itself.

I tell Dr. Gerling: "The patient is a forty-four-year-old man who was doing a gymnastics maneuver on a beam. As he was suspended vertically in the air with his feet straight up, the beam gave way, and he came crashing down on the top of his head. The spine CT was originally read as a fracture of the spinous process of C7 and vertebral body fractures of T5 and T6. The first rib on the right broke as well."

The spinous process is the bulge you feel coming out of your back over the vertebra, C7 refers to the seventh cervical vertebrae, and T stands for thoracic. *Thoracic* is the proper term for *chest*. If you fully fracture the seventh cervical vertebra and if it moves, you are paralyzed from the neck down.

"What was a forty-four-year-old guy doing a gymnastic twirl up in the air like that for?" Dr. Gerling asks.

"Well, it was really on a goal post in a soccer match. The goal post wasn't bolted down. So when the twirl of the body went straight up, the goal post fell over, and the entire weight of the body, two hundred twenty pounds, came crashing down on the top of his head. *Bang!* Like being hit on the top of the head with a sledgehammer." It was just easier to describe it as a gymnastics accident. "Oh, yes, this is a pile-driver injury."

Dr. Gerling and Dr. Onesti look at the films more closely and point out the snapped-off piece of bone in the neck.

Dr. Gerling says, "He snapped off the spinous process of C7. That thing will recalcify like a bandit. He will be normal in six weeks." Another bullet dodged. "Where is the patient?"

"It's me. These are my films."

TWO DAYS BEFORE, I had returned from Ireland, where I'd gone to attend the wedding of my boss's daughter, who happens to be a Pulitzer Prize–winning expert on the history of genocide in the 20th century and a senior foreign policy adviser to then-candidate Barack Obama. Her groom is the owner and operator of perhaps the finest legal mind in the country. On the morning of the wedding, they scheduled an atypical prenuptial event—a soccer game—which was entirely logical given the International guest list. The goalie was from the United Nations Commission on Refugees. The defense opposition included the *New York Times* correspondent for Afghanistan and more members of the United Nations. Our offense had Human Rights Watch and the United States' leading legal expert on election law. The president of Burundi was playing offense for my side. In the audience was the leading war crimes prosecutor for the tribunal at The Hague, a speechwriter for President Kennedy, the director of the film *Hotel Rwanda,* and the dean of Harvard Law School. Here I was with some of the most accomplished people on the planet, feeling like everything I had ever done was so small by comparison. I also had not played soccer in 30 years.

I had no idea what I was doing, and so I substituted drive, enthusiasm, and aggressiveness for actual skill. We were getting our asses kicked, and by the time we finally scored a goal, I was desperate to impress the women. I was seized by the urge to swing my 220-pound, six-foot-four self around the goal post. *Crash!* I came down straight on my head. The goal post also crashed a large steel pole on the back of my neck. I felt and heard a sickly pop in my spine. Numbness and tingling went down both my arms. I didn't move.

"I think I have broken my neck," I said with surprising calm.

So much for showing off. My first thought was *How will I take care of my children if I'm paralyzed from the neck down?* A minute later my boss, Dr. Edmund Bourke, was standing over me. The ambulance was called, and an instant tent of people with umbrellas was standing over me, a shelter from the cold rain of a cloudy Irish morning.

"Dr. Bourke, I just want you to know, since I might not be coming back, that if I do turn out to be paralyzed, I would not have done anything different in my life except for two things."

"What's that, Conrad?"

"I would have prayed more, and danced more."

He looked like he was going to cry.

"I love you, boss." I said. For once, no one thought I was more emotional than events deserved.

I got placed on a stiff backboard, and my head was immobilized. They rolled me as one piece and stabilized my neck, because if there was a neck fracture and my head moved, my spinal cord would be severed, and I'd be dead. On the 45-minute ride to the nearest hospital, I contemplated my weaknesses, especially the ones that had compelled me to show off. Not for one minute did I doubt the care I was in, and as the author of ten medical textbooks, I was the ultimate empowered patient. My faith in the spine surgeon was completely undiminished. The simple trust that bounds us together in the doctor-patient relationship was as vibrant and real as any had ever been.

In the emergency department, a nervous-looking young doctor came instantly to examine me. They rolled me to palpate my spine and see if I could wiggle my toes, which I could.

"Look, Doc," I told him, "you can do whatever you want, but if you can get cervical spine films done in the next ten minutes I would appreciate it. Also, can you CT scan my thoracic spine? I think I broke some vertebrae around T5 and T6."

"Why do you know so much?" he asked. "What do you do?"

I tell him.

Now he was really nervous: "Fine! Go ahead and scare me," he said.

"What's wrong? You're doing fine. Why so nervous?"

He replied: "I am an intern, and I only started working here two days ago."

I had to laugh. "It's okay. Just get me the spine films. You will be fine. I promise I will tell everyone this story when we are done."

"Okay, I also have to do a rectal exam to check for rectal tone."

Now *I* started looking nervous. "I refuse the rectal! Got that? R-e-f-u-s-e, as in no!"

He didn't seem that disappointed, and that was a good thing.

Time stretched. First, the immobility was excruciating. Since I wasn't able to move for an hour, the lactic acid started to accumulate in my muscles, and everything was painful. Second, I was waiting to see if my life as I knew it was finished. No more teaching. No more performing. Just sitting in a wheelchair changing a urinary catheter.

During this time, I was branded with understanding of the importance of my profession. I became acutely aware that help is not available to all, that most Americans are not in the club that receives such VIP care. I made a note to make sure things moved fast in the hospital in the future, which I have had the good fortune to practice to this day.

ALTHOUGH I'D FRACTURED three vertebrae and a rib, my spinal cord was undamaged. I walked out of the hospital.

Back home people were celebrating the Fourth of July, and here I was in Ireland enjoying the greatest freedom of them all—a new lease on life. As an uninsured foreigner, I figured I would get hit for something between $2,000 and $5,000 for the costs of the multiple physician evaluations, the ambulance ride, the many X-rays, and the CT scan. I was stunned to get a bill for 187 euros, or, at the time, about $250. This means for the 47 million uninsured Americans, it would be cheaper to fly to Europe for care than to be seen in a U.S. emergency department.

I renewed my commitment to universal coverage back home. I decided to write a book of stories about the abundant good that modern medicine can do. My aim in writing this book has been to inspire doctors and patients, voters and legislators, to seize the moment and bring about universal coverage, an idea whose time has surely come. Making the treatments covered in these pages a matter of routine for every American is not only within our grasp but would be our greatest miracle yet.

In the midst of an economic crisis, President Barack Obama has astonished even a die-hard optimist like me by keeping his campaign promise to drive straight on ahead to solve some of the thorniest issues of health care: financing, research, and restoring science to its proper place in the society, one that is free of politics. What is my part in this? To inoculate the best and brightest of our society against negativity, false despair, and fear. To attract them to the president's extraordinary endeavor. To shield their minds from a rampant cynicism and narrow-mindedness of senior physicians and faculty and to inspire them to get back in that laboratory and find cures—for cancer, for rheumatoid arthritis, for asthma, for blindness, for depression, and for myriad other causes of suffering.

The best minds of our generation will need positivity and optimism, unlimited energy and enthusiasm. And they will need the confident hope that when you gather the smartest people in the room in the search for a cure, they will find it.

NOTE ABOUT THE INTERVIEWS

THIS BOOK IS NOT an even work. It does not devote equal time to each specialty or even try to touch every one. It aims to capture the spirit of discovery through a selection of remarkable advances in order to inspire the current crop of graduates to pursue research careers and bring hope to patients who are waiting for cures. Originally I had planned to look at advances throughout the country, but I found so many amazing things in my own backyard that I rarely traveled outside Brooklyn. Because there are many world-class people at the State University of New York Health Sciences Center at Brooklyn (SUNY Downstate) and because it is a university training program, most of the patients and experts I interviewed are at Downstate.

I have gone to considerable lengths to protect privacy in this book. Patients have provided both verbal and written consent for the use of their stories. The interview process was approved by an institutional review board (IRB). By itself, the IRB is an advance that would fit in well with the theme of this book, except that it is not new: it is a 50-year-old response to the horrors of involuntary experimentation during World War II and infamous ethical lapses such as the Tuskegee syphilis studies. The IRB makes sure that each participant knows what the study is for, what will be done with the information, and what all the risks and benefits of the study are. An IRB must include scientists and physicians as well as ethicists and members of the community. They are an independent group of people with no benefit in the outcome of the study that makes sure the study is fair, humane, well-explained, and noncoercive. Today no one can publish data in the scientific and medical literature without proof of IRB approval. The IRB at my institution took months of review and numerous revisions to ensure that everyone you read about in this book was spoken to in a proper manner about his or her condition.